The Scents of Health

A User-Friendly Guide to Aromatherapy

By L. Carl Robinson

Steven H. Horne, Editor

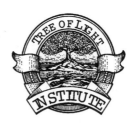

About the Tree of Light Institute: The Tree of Light
Institute is an independent educational organization dedicated to
research, writing, and education in the field of natural health,
focusing on herbs and nutrition. We publish two bimonthly
journals called *Nature's Field: A Journal of Holistic Healing,* and
Healing Light: Your Natural Friend. In addition to this, we have
several correspondence courses and other publications that focus
on natural healing. For more information on our products and
services, please write or call: Tree of Light Institute, P.O. Box
1028, Roosevelt, UT 84066, (435) 722-5080.

Disclaimer: The information in this booklet is **for
educational purposes only.** Always consult with a qualified
health practitioner before deciding on any course of treatment,
especially for serious or life-threatening illnesses. The Tree of
Light Institute is an independent publishing company and does
not receive support from any manufacturer of herbs or
nutritional supplements.

ISBN # 1-890855-08-1

Table of Contents

Introduction

Over fifteen years ago, I was introduced to aromatherapy while in the process of obtaining a Master Herbalist degree in herbal pharmacology/ pharmocognosy. Part of my studies included a segment on a dozen or so essential oils, which were major components of some of the herbs covered in that course. After finishing my studies I began developing herbal formulas for various companies (many of which are still in the market place) and specific tisane (teas) formulations for my growing clientele.

I don't really know what impelled me to take a closer look at essential oils and the field of aromatherapy. Maybe it was my youthful obsession with having a fine collection of men's toiletries and fragrances. At one point I had over 40 different fragrances from around the world in my collection. Mind you, I'm not talking of cheap AquaVelva™ or Mennon™ stuff. I'm talking of men's fragrances from the finest perfume and fragrance houses of Europe. Long ago, I pared that collection down to a couple of dozen or so, but I still enjoy fragrances.

Or perhaps it's my obsession with having a whole kitchen cupboard full of spices and cooking herbs, most of which are aromatic. Let's see, last count I think there were over three dozen, and that's the single dried herbs and spices only! The average American kitchen has only eight such seasonings in their cupboard of which salt and pepper are two. I've even heard of silly attempts to consider table sugar a spice.

Whatever the underlying reason, I have spent over fifteen years of my professional life researching the use of essential oils. Part of my work has been groundbreaking research and practical application of essential oils for internal nutritional-therapeutic use. This endeavor has been fascinating and oftentimes surprising. In addition, I have utilized aromatherapy in my hypnotherapy practice. The results have been just as fascinating.

It is in that same spirit that I suspect you are reading this book. For indeed, aromatic essential oils, which I refer to throughout this guide as EO's, are fascinating. They represent what is still a fairly exotic area of phyto-botanical lore and science and everyone knows that the more exotic something is, the more curious we tend to be about it.

As for the surprising part, get ready for one of the most exciting experiences in herbalism and natural healing there is. EO's are some of the most subtle, yet profound biological substances we can use to improve our health and wellbeing, especially where emotional and neurological wellbeing are concerned.

This book is written in what I call 'chunk-style.' A lot of information will be shared with you in concise fashion without taking up volumes of pages. With that said, sit back, blow your nose and clear your head to get it ready for all those great smells and sensations, and enjoy the exotic, sensuous and healing world of aromatic essential oils.

L. Carl Robinson

Chapter One

The History of Aromatherapy

The sense of smell is one of the most primal of all our senses. It extends back to the time when humans needed this sense for survival, as a means of smelling some wild animal lurking around the corner or knowing the scent of edible or poisonous plants. What the ancient man hoped for was that he had not been 'smelled-out' by the wild animal itself, who's sense of smell was usually far keener than humans. From this awareness of odor, humans learned how to hunt dangerous animals by being aware of the time of day, temperature, season, and the ever-present direction of breeze flow. If the breeze was blowing face-wards into the hunter, his scent would blow away from his quarry, making it easier to stalk and take. However, if the direction of breeze changed and blew from his back towards the animal, his own life was then in peril.

Becoming Aware of Smell's Affects

As humans became more aware of the plants that grew about them (hence a rudimentary herbology) they also noted a peculiar thing about these plants. When they flowered, or exuded a resin or exudate, there was a smell that accompanied the event. Even more interesting to these early humans were the different feelings they had when smelling these aromas.

Some plant aromas made them feel relaxed or sedated. Others made them perk up and feel refreshed, invigorated or more aware of their surroundings. On the other hand some of the plant exudates gave off pungent putrid smells, almost akin to that of death. These smells were nauseating, and often might make them feel dizzy, disoriented or just plain scarred. These aromas helped human beings to determine the qualities of a plant, whether it was good for food or medicine, or poisonous, much the same as animals use their noses for the same purpose today.

Thus, to our ancestors, smell was the primary means of establishing the safety or danger of a substance or the environment. Even today, where we don't know the safety of something, we often use our sense of smell as the primary determinant for safety or danger.

Egyptian Unguents & Incense

The written history of aromatic essential oils and their earliest specific uses come from the first dynasties of Egypt. There are hieroglyphs that show people applying unguents to each other. An unguent is a fatty based salve to which aromatic plants were covered and allowed to sit for a number of weeks. After this period the fat was separated from the plant material and the resulting salve-like substance was the now scented unguent. Small clay vessels have been found in the ancient tombs of Egypt that contain traces of these aromatic unguents. Myrrh gum, frankincense, cedar and other aromas derived from plants growing along the Nile and from other areas of

Africa and the Middle East have been detected. The sun-king Akhnaton (1370-1352 BCE) built the city of Akhenaton (Tel-el-Amarna) which was built with hygiene being its first consideration. Along with its decree that only clean water be allowed into the city and that all 'brown' water be immediately removed was a law mandating that piles of smudges (a rudimentary form of incense) prepared from aromatic herbs and plants be burnt in the public squares daily to cleanse and purify the air of the city.

India, Ayurveda and Poor-Man's Medicine

Late Drivadian and early Indo-European sub-continent India also record similar uses and applications for aromatic unguents.

Over the centuries the various cultures of the world, to one degree or another, learned how to use specific herbs and spices in their foods and developed unique culinary traditions. India (with its Ayurvedic system of medicine) developed a whole sub-category of therapy around the culinary usage of herbs and spices indigenous to their area. In fact, many indigenous societies still resort to their "poor-man's" medicine chest that consists of nothing more than a few culinary herbs and spices. These are used in foods to both prevent and cure illness, often with profound and effective results.

Persian Alchemists

To ascertain the first substantiated use of pure aromatic essential oils our history tour next takes us to the middle Persian Empire and their alchemists.

The Persian alchemists were gifted as to their scientific thinking and abilities. While Europe was in the superstitious mire of the Middle Ages, the Persians were at the zenith of their culture. Their science, based on advanced mathematical concepts, was considered the most advanced of the time. Their knowledge and understanding of astronomy even without the use of a telescope, was unsurpassed because of the accuracy of their mathematical calculations.

By historical standards their medicine was also very advanced. Many of the Persian alchemists were cross-trained in various fields, which gave them a unique eclectic view of life and its workings. A holistic approach indeed. No where was this of more help than in understanding the aromatic components of plants and how to distill the 'spirit' of the plant into its pure form. Thus, they became the first people we know of to actually distill pure aromatic oils from plants.

By astute observation, the Persian alchemist learned that the unseen aroma of a plant, which they referred to as its spirit, was actually something real. They concluded this, based on the observation that smell was a physical phenomenon, and the fact that certain scents had a specific affect on emotions and physiological responses.

Discovery of Distillation

The high point in their observations came when they began to note that only at certain times in a plant's development, and more importantly only during certain times of the day, were they able to detect the plant's aroma. They ascertained that as a general rule when the sun was an hour or two from its zenith the plant released the highest level of aroma. This is the point when the coolness of the morning turns to the heat of the afternoon. In this observation lay the key to their theorizing the process of distillation.

They concluded, and rightly so, that a mild sort of transitional heat needed to be applied to the plant to release its "spirit." Using common sense and some creative experimentation they were able to develop what we call a 'goose neck' apparatus for distilling the aromatic components of a plant. By today's standards it was crude, but back then it was a state-of-art piece of equipment. One of the theories these alchemists had was that if the heat was just low enough it would impel the plant to give up it spirit in pure form. If the heat went too high it would next cause the water to boil and therefore infiltrate the distillate. Through tedious experimentation they proved their theory correct and the basic tenants of distillation, which are still used to this day, were born.

Then, as today, a plants aromatic oils were derived from whole plants, flowers, citrus peels, trees, bark and roots. These oils were called "spirits" or "essences" because they were thought to actually be the spirit or essence of the plant. These concepts remain in our language today as we refer to distilled alcoholic beverages as "spirits" and aromatherapy oils as "essential" oils.

Perfume Trade

From this effort was born the Persian perfume trade. It spread like wildfire throughout the Middle East, the Indian sub-continent (which was by now under Islamic rule) and the greater Orient. Then, by way of Istanbul (Constantinople) it made its way into Europe.

History has it that the Queen of Hungary (a country which was partly under Muslim rule) was given a 'toilet water' as a gift. It consisted of citrus and spice aromatic essential oils mixed in a stable mixture of water and grain alcohol. This toiletry came to be known as 'Hungary Water.' It was an immediate sensation with the royal courts of Europe. The king of France was so impressed with it that he chartered the first perfumery house of Europe, the House of Farina, to exclusively manufacture perfumes for the King and his royal court. It was a blend, still in existence today, similar to Hungary Water, except a bit spicier. Last I heard, the House of Farina was still in existence and doing a booming business.

Going back to the Persians, their doctors, especially the Sufi masters who were gifted healers, developed an extensive protocol for the use of various types of pure essential oils as healing and calming agents. This they did by applying the oils to pulse points and joints of the body. Important places they applied these oils included: behind the ears, over the eyebrows, along the jaw line, on the wrists and ankles, and on the soft areas of the knees and elbows. We'll talk more about this in the therapeutic section of this book. Even today, many of the most successful uses of aromatic essential oils relative to emotional healing are based on the ancient Sufi healing traditions developed centuries ago.

The Great Plagues

The Middle East is not the only place where the therapeutic benefits of essential oils were experienced. One of the most famous stories concerning the use of aromatic plants as preventative health agents is the "Four Thieves of Paris." At the height of the Great Plague, which riddled the Middle East and then Europe, there were four men that worked during the day at a place that made aromatic vinegar. Their firm used aromatic plants (such as juniper, marjoram, sage, wormwood, rosemary, etc.). During the night these four men would stalk the diseased places of Paris and steal the valuables of the sick and dying. They did this with complete immunity to the plague. During one of their evening forays these men were caught and brought to trial for their crimes. What perplexed the court was how they, and no one else, could move among the sick and dying without becoming ill. The answer is that they had partaken of a vinegar extract of aromatic herbs (and had also handled all of those aromatic herbs throughout the day). The story has it they traded their vinegar recipe in exchange for a reduced sentence.[1] The highly disinfectant and antiseptic

---

[1] The event actually took place during the great plagues that affected Toulouse, France (1628 – 1631). The Parliament of Toulouse's archives record that: "During the great plague, four

nature of the aromatic compounds in the herbs had protected these men from the great bubonic plague.

There are similar, but less known stories, about aromatics being used in the Great Plague. I've been told that the Sufi healing masters and Persian manufacturers of aromatic oils were also left untouched during the great plagues of the Middle East. Also, in India during outbreaks of plague those who dealt in aromatic spices and herbs were immune to the effects of this deadly disease as well.

Of Liquors, Meads and Digestifs

Eventually aromatic plants were used extensively by the European monks to make their honey meads, digestifs and medicinal liquors. Many of these meads and liquors still commercially exist today, being sold as flavored liquors. Familiar names such as Benedictine, Chartreuse, Sambuca and Jaggermeister are all popular flavored liquors today that were originally developed as medicinal agents for digestive disorders, wasting, respiratory conditions, etc.

(Speaking of liquors and their use of highly aromatic plants, I might here add that the aromatic components of a plant are no less important than that of a fine wine's vintage. Factors such as how much

robbers were convicted of going to the houses of plague-victims, strangling them in their beds and then looting their dwellings; for this they were condemned to be burned at the stake, and in order to have the sentence mitigated they revealed their secret preservative; after which they were hanged."

tannins, sugars, minerals, etc all contribute to the uniqueness of every wine, but it's the subtle aromatic components that give the wine its complexity. Things such as 'bouquet,' whether is has a 'berry' or 'floral' nose, along with a plethora of other terms describe the aroma qualities of a wine. In fact, the most trusted apparatus for detecting the aroma quality of a wine is... you got it! The nose.)

This brings the history of using essential oils up to modern times. Both the food flavoring and designer perfumery trade have long used aromatic oils for cosmetic and food flavoring purposes. In fact, up until just ten years ago, the majority of the world's supply of aromatic oils was used in these two industries. However, there was also a great deal of research into the uses of these oils taking place in the background, especially in France, Germany and Italy. Not since the middle Persian Empire has the same creative and studious efforts been put into the distilling[2], blending

---

[2]Generally, quality aromatic oils result from a double distillation process that's referred to as 'Standard' in the industry. The highest quality aromatic essential oils are derived from triple distillation and are referred to as 'Extra.' Triple distilled substantially increases the end cost and is often required by the perfume trade. Some of the 'extra' EO's also used for therapeutic use are Lavender, Geranium, Bergamot, Rose and Ylang Ylang. For therapeutic use relative to topical and nutritional therapy, the standard distilled EO's are more than adequate, excepting the previously mentioned 'Extra' EO's. Single distilled EO's which are derived from passing steam through culinary herbs and spices (of which the depleted herbs and spices are then sold to an unsuspecting consumer) are most often used for food flavoring in the foods industry. They are

and therapeutic uses of aromatic essential oils. The West is now making its own unique contributions to the world of Essential Oils.

---

generally unacceptable for therapeutic use due to their high content of sediment and impurities.

Chapter Two

The Biology of Aromatherapy

Essential oils have a specific affinity for the nerve tissues of the body. The most immediate point of nerve contact is that of the olfactory membranes located in the sinus cavity. These membranes contain the nerve endings that are responsible for the sense of smell. These nerves connect directly to a part of our brain known as the olfactory bulb, which has direct connections to many other areas of the mind.

One of these connections is to the hypothalamus, the stalk of the brain that controls the pituitary gland, which controls, in turn, the rest of the glandular system of the body. Thus, aromatherapy is being shown to have a powerful impact on our endocrine system. Aromatherapy oils can relieve menstrual irregularities, enhance energy and even sexual desire.

The sense of smell is also intimately connected to that part of the brain called the limbic area, the area of memory. The limbic area deals with responses like fight or flight, pain and pleasure and perceptions of bad and good. One thing for sure, the limbic area is intimately involved with the sub-conscious. Here we see that the sense of smell also has an immediate and powerful impact on both memory and emotion (Hypnotherapists know what implications this has). Perhaps this is why we say, "the nose knows."

The Subjective Nature of Aroma

In the mid 1980's I read an issue of the *National Geographic* dedicated to the sense of smell and the then fast growing field of 'Aromatherapy.' Although I enjoyed reading the scientific and industrial information about aromatherapy, I was particularly intrigued with the lead writer's introduction.

He recalled an earlier assignment for the *National Geographic* where he and his photographer assistant went to a Midwest-type community. Having just finished breakfast, they headed out on the day's assignment. Exiting the premises, as they stood on the porch, the smell of freshly laid asphalt and tar wafted their way. The road in front of where they had stayed had just been paved while they were enjoying breakfast.

His assistant immediately closed her eyes and recalled how that smell reminded her so much of her young childhood. It brought back memories of the good times—the friends, fun and idyllic summers of her childhood, when every summer the town's road crew would pass somewhere in her neighborhood and lay a new asphalt surface. For her, the aroma of the tar evoked a wonderful flood of pleasant memories.

The author's experience was quite different. For him the smell of the asphalt and tar brought up melancholy and feelings of sadness. In fact, it put him into a deep state of depression. As a young boy he used to spend his summers working with his dad, who was a roofer. Asphalt shingles and hot tar were a daily part of their work. One day, while working on an extremely steep roof, his dad slipped on a patch of tar. He was unable to stop himself from sliding down the roof and fell to his death breaking his neck when he hit the ground. As a young boy the author witnessed this tragedy, the smell of asphalt and roofing tar strong in his nostrils.

For the lady photographer the aroma of tar aroused fond memories of a pleasurable childhood. For the author, the same aroma prompted an instant intense recall of one of the most tragic moments in his life.

This story illustrates a vital point, one of the most important in dealing with the therapeutic use of aromatic essential oils or EO's. (From here on throughout this guide I will use the acronym **EO's** interchangeably with the word aromatic essential oils.) The sense of smell and its extremely powerful effect on memory makes the emotional responses invoked by particular oil highly subjective. While one fragrance might be pleasant and uplifting to the majority of people, for others that same aroma might bring painful memories to the awareness, thus invoking a depressing response. Hence, the exact effect of an EO can vary greatly from individual to individual.

I've seen this phenomenon numerous times in my work as a clinical herbalist and clinical hypnotherapist. The therapeutic or neuro-emotional usage of an EO or its emotional effect as listed in this book (or any other book for that matter) is purely a 'general' reference. Never forget the subjective aspect of aromatherapy when a person does not respond exactly as a reference says they should.

Neurological Differences

Added to the subjective nature of individual memories invoked by various aromas is the fact that everyone's nervous system (neurology) is different. Hence, even our conditioned physio-emotional responses to various stimuli differ. Permit me to share a personal account of how these differences worked in the actual marketplace.

In the late 1980's I developed two unique aromatic mineral tonic products. Each contained a complex blend of EO's in a base of liquid trace minerals (LTM's). I had extensively used these two components (the LTM's and the EO's) separately in practice in my therapy center. These products were the first of their kind in the health products industry. No one had previously developed, for the general consumer, essential oil formulas for internal therapeutic use.

Having already gained extensive clinical experience in the internal therapeutic usage of EO's, I designed these products around two basic nervous system types. My premise was based on working with the two branches of the autonomic nervous system, the sympathetic and the parasympathetic. These two aspects of our autonomic nervous system lie at the root of all physiological and emotional responses in the body. The two types are the sympathetic and parasympathetic. The sympathetic type is a "type A" or "yang" type. They tend to be active, mobile and otherwise "on the go." The parasympathetic type is a "type B" or "yin" personality, more relaxed, settled and "laid back."

I had already spent a number of years in literary and clinical research on the effects of essential oils. At that time literature on the subject was limited, but in the interim I had acquired a great deal of practical experience. I had blended oils for individuals in my therapy center (which was located in a medical plaza) and had observed the overall effects of different EO's on my clients.

I was literally breaking new ground on this one. I came to realize this because I had been ordering oils from and directly collaborating with three of the largest distiller/manufacturers of EO's in the world, who told me they were not aware of anyone working on using EO's in this manner. I felt like a real pioneer at the time.

When I developed the aforementioned aromatic mineral tonic products, one was developed to enhance sympathetic responses of the nervous system and the other to enhance parasympathetic responses. To put it in simpler terms, one product was designed to enliven the body via the sympathetic nervous system, while the other was designed to relax the body via the parasympathetic responses.

When I did preliminary tests and limited market provings the products seemed to work just as I expected. However, when I took the product into the greater marketplace I got some incongruent results.

Though most people responded to the products just as I had expected, there were also many individuals who experienced the exact opposite response. In other words, among a fairly large segment of those consuming the products the neuro-physiological response to the products was as expected, but there was also a number of individuals upon whom these products worked in the opposite direction. At first this really concerned me, but I held off making any knee-jerk reactions or snap judgements and continued to observe what was happening.

What I discovered was that everyone who used both of the products did experience the two differing neuro-physiological responses. What was happening was that those who were responding differently responded backwards from the majority of people. You see, there were a percentage of people who had a parasympathetic response from the sympathetic blend and a sympathetic response to the parasympathetic formula.

My conclusions were that some people respond exactly opposite of others with various essential oils. The upshot is this: *Be very careful when using any EO's therapeutically (especially internal) as the subjective response of the therapy can vary from individual to individual, even when using the exact same blend and regime.* This does not mean they are responding wrongly or that the EO is bad, it just means that a person's neurological polarity is reversed from that of other people.

There are some very good EO products and blends on the market; however, realize that what the blend may be "indicated" for, it may actually aggravate. Conversely, something an EO is normally "contraindicated" for it may actually help in certain individuals. It's not that the single oil or blend is bad or wrong in and of itself (though some are poorly formulated or just plain outright poor quality). It's just that we're dealing with the subtle peculiarities and idiosyncratic nature of the nervous system and the variations such idiosyncratic phenomena elicit from person to person.

The "Holistic Effect" of EO's

When I was doing my research, most of the literature and reference work I was accessing was based on the germ theory of Pasteur. Most of the research dealt with the "anti" actions of the oils, such as antibiotic, antiseptic or antiparasitic. Though there were correlations between my work and the research I'd referenced to, none of the research addressed the neuro-physiological aspects of EO's usage, at least not to the degree I was addressing it. In those early years the literature was also very limited in addressing the subtle emotional responses that result from using aromatic essential oils.

Realizing this, I stepped back and reassessed the landscape of what I was doing. In this manner I was able to ascertain a very important principle of EO's and their usage. I realized that I was operating more from Beauchamp's holistic terrain theory of the pleomorphic[3] cause of disease rather than Pasteur's isolate germ theory of the monomorphic[4] cause of disease.

The literature stated that EO's have an extremely high affinity for nerve tissue. The brain, brain stem and spinal column are all nerve tissue. The research

---

[3] The 'Pleomorphic' theory of disease causation as elucidated by Antoine Beauchamp, M.D. stated that all forms of disease arose out of one universal germ entity, and that the metamorphic action of changing from one disease to another (with its resultant effects) could only ensue if the appropriate medium and environment were present for a specific aspect of the universal germ to manifest itself. This theory was validated in the 'light refracting' microscopic work of William Rife, M.D. through a specially constructed microscope that used dark-field condenensers he had developed in which the actual metamorphisis of germs were observed to actually happen. This important work with its life saving potential, like Beauchamp's holistic view of disease processes, was vigorously opposed, suppressed and eventually destroyed by the pharmaceutical interests and prevailing medical orthodoxy of the day.

[4] The 'Monomorphic' theory of disease causation as elucidated by Louis Pasteur, M.D. stated that all disease was caused by specific germs that exherted a specific effect on the medium they were placed in contact with. All modern pharmacy and medicine exists and rests on this theory. The problem is that this theory is based on a purely in-vitro approach, the test tube. Unlike pleomorphism, monomorphism has never stood the rigorous standards of in-vivo research. Even as recently as 1983, two eminent cancer fellowship research doctors of the Pasteur Institute, Sorin Sonea, & Maurice Panisset boldly proclaimed to the world in their book *A New Bacteriology* (Jones & Bartlett, Boston, 1983) that Beauchamp (and his pleomorphic theory) was correct and had been from the beginning.

literature also showed that nerves function in a rhythmic fashion, like a pendulum, meaning they run in cycles every hour, day, month and season of the year. These cycles are like flows of energy. From this I learned there is polarity in all of this, meaning a given charge of energy, say a negative one, will result in a given response, whereas another given charge of energy, say a positive one, will result in a different (usually opposite) given response. It's that simple! Or so I thought.

As mentioned earlier, the sense of smell is intimately connected to that part of the brain called the limbic area, the area of memory. Here is where both memory and its attendant emotional responses are triggered. A knowledge of the role that the limbic area plays in triggering emotional responses by memory reflex is absolutely essential to those who do *Neuro-Associative Processing (NAP)*. This is now popularized term I coined over 15 years ago. It also plays a role in the varying types of emotional release work.

From a hypnotherapy point of view (which often utilizes NAP) this has incredibly broad ramifications. Hypnotherapy (and all other types of qualified emotional healing work) operates on the premise that healing is accomplished by clarifying, overcoming and changing self-defeating and dysfunctional behavior. Thus, "negative" behavior is replaced with functionally healthy behavior through a discovery of the underlying belief systems and values that drive a person's emotions. These belief systems and their resultant values are embedded into the neurological makeup (the memory) of every individual causing them to react to people and situations in a particular and often predictable way.

Once a person understands the belief systems and resultant values which govern the way they behave in given situations and circumstances, they can use this new found clarity to consciously chose to change these belief systems. Because it helps to access deeply held feelings and memories aromatherapy can be very beneficial in this type of work. In my own practice of hypnotherapy, which extensively incorporates NAP, I help to reinforce the follow through of a person's changes through aromatherapy (as well as herbs, nutrition and lifestyle changes).

Synthetic versus Natural

EO's are fragile complex hydrocarbon molecules that consist of various combinations of alcohols, esters, benzines, camphors, aldehydes, terpines, phenols, and a host of other carbon based components. Some EO's will contain a higher proportion of aldehydes and phenols (such as mints), while others will be higher in esters, and terpines (such as the citrus EO's). It is the complex chemical configurations of these hydrocarbon components that give each oil its unique aroma and properties.

Due to their extremely complex chemical makeup many EO's have not been synthesized in the laboratory. Those scents that have been synthetically reproduced do not exhibit the same therapeutic response as the natural EO's do. This is because the polarization of the synthetic is always the opposite of the natural, and hence results in the opposite therapeutic effect.

Take lavender oil for instance. Whereas natural lavender oil has an anti-inflammatory action on tissues, the synthesized lavender oil has an inflammatory action on tissues.

There is a well repeated story in aromatherapy circles that comes out of Europe where a business traveler who had an inflamed condition of the colon was on an extended business trip and ran out of lavender oil. His doctor had him topically applying the oil to reduce the swelling and inflammation of his condition. He went to a local chemist (pharmacy in the U.S.) to buy a bottle of lavender oil. At his hotel he applied the oil as he had always done. Instead of cooling and reducing the inflammation of his condition, his tissues were burning and swelling. At the hospital they had to take emergency measures to correct the situation. Upon reviewing what had happened it was discovered that the chemist had sold him a bottle of synthetic lavender oil, not the natural variety he had always bought before. This is a classical example of natural versus synthetic.

This same phenomenon is observed in virtually every EO that's ever been chemically synthesized. Vanilla, lemon, mints, cinnamon, clove, pine and thyme are just a few of the oils chemists have attempted to copy from nature and have consistently fallen short of as to their therapeutic value. Many of the isolated and chemically synthesized components of EO's, (such as phenols, used for antiseptic and antibacterial purposes) also fall short of the benefits found in using the whole and natural EO's from which they are derived.

In fact, the phenolic-based antiseptic cleaners used in hospitals no longer kill the super staph germs prevalent in American hospitals. These super-germs are now immune to the isolated components of EO's, but not to the whole EO itself. In Europe where the use of whole aromatic essential oils as disinfecting agents is common, there is no problem with those same super-germs. Most European hospitals are more holistically inclined than American hospitals are. Hmm. Could it be that they are enjoying better health care as a result?

Scientific Research on EO's

On a scientific level from research coming out of Europe EO's have been well documented as to their effects on bacteria, viruses, fungus, molds and other germs, as well as the cleansing effect they have upon the air.

Have you ever been in a eucalyptus grove or in the pine forest of a mountain? Did you notice how refreshing the air was? In each of these instances, the trees were giving off aromatic components that had the effect of ionizing the air about them. That's right! Certain EO's have the effect of ionizing and refreshing the air. That's why in many hospitals throughout Europe, especially in France, a nebulizing aromatherapy diffuser is used to disinfect and clean the air. It should be noted that European hospitals that use this means of air purification do not experience the airborne super staph germs that are also rampant in American hospitals.

EO's are extremely sensitive to sunlight (especially the ultra-violet spectrum) and air. The action of the sun causes an EO to break down. Open exposure to air causes the lighter components, say the alcohols, to evaporate from the EO, thereby altering the character of the EO as the heavier components, like terpines and phenols, begin to concentrate. This alters the purity, character and therapeutic integrity of an EO. Air, with its oxygen content, also causes an oxidative process to ensue which itself dramatically reduces the purity and effectiveness of an EO.

Research also exists on the topical use of EO's and their effects on the physiology and emotions of people. However, this form of research is more subjective and traditional. But, everyone, including the scientific community, should remember that this is the oldest therapeutic use of EO's. Hence, the use of oils for settling the emotions is one that has stood the test of time. Many popular massage and bodywork products are formulated upon the generally accepted emotional responses to particular blends of EO's. Some of these blends are based on formulas that are many generations old.

Testing the Effects of EO's

As mentioned earlier, EO's have a specific affinity for the nerve tissues of the body. The most immediate point of nerve contact is that of the olfactory glands in the sinus cavity. As the aroma of the EO makes contact with the olfactory nerve endings there is a distinct neuro-chemical response that takes place in the brain. This response almost always results in some sort of neuro-associatively driven memory reflex throughout the body, that's usually first felt in the solar plexus of the body. The immediate solar plexus response will usually be a relaxed settling one or an acrid uptight squeezing feeling. This is the first indicator of whether an EO or EO's blend is compatible with the body (and emotions) at that point in time.

I have found that the smell/taste approach to determining which EO's to use or recommend is also quite effective. In some systems that use a smell/taste response testing method it is assumed that if it smells or tastes bad then the body needs it. In aromatherapy the premise is that if it smells or tastes bad then it should not be given to the body. Conversely, if it smells or tastes good, the body needs it.

Because of the profound effect EO's have on the neuro-emotional responses of the body, it is important to select oils which cause a positive neuro-associative response. When selecting oils, let yourself or your client smell the fragrances, paying particular attention to how the aroma makes them feel in the region of the solar plexus. (This is the soft spot just under the breastbone and at the top of the abdominal cavity.)

Solar Plexus Response Testing

If the oil makes the solar plexus relax (which usually results in a calmer feeling and more relaxed deep breathing), then the oil is having a positive effect on the individual. If the solar plexus tightens and the person's experience of the oils is one of tension and unpleasantness, that oil is not right for the individual.

Each EO has an overall specific effect upon the neurological makeup of a person. And as mentioned earlier, it can vary from individual to individual. I've found that all emotional responses can be narrowed down to four basic physiological reactions. It is from various combinations of these four basic reactions that the myriad "shades" and "colors" of emotional responses arise. The four physio-emotional effects are expansive (relaxing), contractive (tensing), sedating (calming) and activating (stimulating). Let me elaborate on this.

As we previously discussed, the body's autonomic nervous system has two parts, the sympathetic branch and the parasympathetic branch. The autonomic nervous system gets its name because it operates automatically, without conscious thought or effort on our part. It's what runs all the organ systems of our body – heart beat, digestion, blood pressure, breathing, swallowing reflex, blinking of the eyes, etc.

However, in spite of the fact that we do not have conscious think to get this part of our nervous system to work, we do have some conscious control, albeit limited, over the workings of this system. For example, when a child throws a temper tantrum and holds their breath they are consciously controlling a function of the autonomic nervous system. But I did say this is a limited ability because if they continue this behavior they will eventually black out and return to normal breathing. This is because the autonomic nervous system overrides the conscious waking tantruming of the child. Only by utilizing a trance like state (as is used in guided imagery or clinical hypnosis) can we access the sub-conscious level of the mind that guides and controls the autonomic nervous system and effect positive beneficial changes to its function.

The sympathetic nervous system is the activating part of the autonomic nervous system. It is responsible for the fight or flight response that happens when reacting to fear or danger, or something as simple as having to meet a deadline at work. It is responsible for extraneous related activity such as work, critical thinking, driving, sports, running, etc. It is akin to the Yang principle. According to the four physio-emotional response basics, the sympathetic responses are contractive and activating. They tense and stimulate the body.

The parasympathetic nervous system is the relaxing part of the autonomic nervous system. It is responsible for the "hey, sit back and relax. Kick your feet up and take a deep breath. Ahh, sigh... etc." It is responsible for introspective related activity such as resting, reflective thinking, meditation, digestion, healing of tissues, etc. It is akin to the Yin principle.

According to the four physio-emotional response basics, the parasympathetic responses are expansive and calming. They slow body function, relax tension and tonify soft muscle activity.

However, these responses in and of themselves are never absolute or arbitrary in living beings. There is a dynamic interaction between these responses in the body, so there is seldom a straight sympathetic or parasympathetic response, except in dire emergencies. Thus, we usually have a combination of sympathetic and parasympathetic actions that combine to create the four basic categories of physio-emotional responses. One of these basic four responses will tend to dominate over the others but they will all be present and active in an interactive way.

For instance, if a person were feeling expansive and activated one would need to determine which is dominant. If the feeling of expansiveness is dominant then the autonomic response can be ascertained as being predominately parasympathetic. If a person were more activated or stimulated then they would be predominately sympathetic. The same holds for a contractive and calm response. If a contractive or tense feeling was dominant then it would be predominately a sympathetic response. Whereas the calm feeling would indicate the parasympathetic was the primary response. It is the predominant effect that determines if a response is largely sympathetic or parasympathetic.

Now, if we go back to the solar plexus, we can see why the solar plexus is a good indicator of what the response of the autonomic nervous system will be to a given influence, such as an EO. By paying attention to this spot on our body (the home of what we call "gut instinct") we can tell what the overall general reaction will be to a given aroma. Does the EO being smelled cause the solar plexus to predominately respond in an expansive, contractive, calming or activating manner?

When using solar plexus response testing, it works best if the individual being tested relaxes before trying to test a particular EO. A short meditation or guided imagery session prior to the testing helps relax and prepare an individual be able to sense these effects more clearly in their body. It is surprising how quick and accurate this form of testing can be in determining the overall neuro-emotional effect an EO will have on a given person's body.

Rudimentary Pulse Diagnoses

Another way to ascertain the effect of an EO on the body is through a rudimentary pulse diagnoses. It is one of my favorites. Did you know that it's a standard procedure in medicine for a doctor to have a patient test their pulse rate anytime they eat a food they may have a sensitivity to? If their pulse speeds up or goes erratic its because they are experiencing an allergic reaction somewhere in or throughout their body. In using the pulse we are not diagnosing a disease or pathological problem. We are sensing the degree of tension or relaxation, stimulation or sedation of the system as indicated through the pulse. This falls well within the scope of "structure and function" claims for alternative health care that federal legislation has made legal and FDA regulations must now comply with. Thus, when used correctly, pulse diagnosis may be employed without crossing over the legal boundary into practicing medicine without a license.

To do a rudimentary pulse diagnosis, first take a baseline pulse of the individual. Note four things. The rate of the pulse per minute[5], the consistency of the pulse, the strength of the pulse, and the duration of the pulse. For effective rudimentary pulse diagnoses these four things must always be taken into account.

Having established a baseline of the pulse rate per, you are then going to go ahead and continue taking the pulse while allowing the person to smell an EO or an EO blend. Note any changes? Does the

---

[5] My training in pulse diagnoses comes from traditional Tibetan medicine practice and although it teaches that one should ascertain the pulse rate based on the pulse taker's (the physician/therapist himself) own full breath cycle I have found in a clinical setting that the high degree of subjectivity found in this part of the practice is unacceptable, especially when the more objective approach of timing the pulse to that of a clock brings more accuracy and consistency to the art itself. Therefore, I recommend the use of a clock (or watch) to ascertain the rate of the pulse. Oriental/Eastern medicine traditions have much to offer in lost knowledge and long standing results, but there are times when even the East must give way to a better, more consistent technique regardless of whether it comes from east or west. Besides, consistency is one of the halmarks of the healers art, and nothing is more consistent and objective than the watch's tick.

pulse rate increase or decrease? Does it stay consistent or does it go erratic? Does the strength of the pulse increase or decrease and does the duration of the pulse shorten or lengthen?

As a general rule, if the pulse remains fairly stable in beats per minute, also stays consistent and does not go erratic, becomes slightly stronger and of moderately longer duration, then the EO being tested is going to have an overall good effect on an individual. Here again, there are going to be variations in the rudimentary pulse diagnoses. It will take practice to get it down. In general, however, you are feeling to see if the pulse "balances" out. One can learn a great deal about the subtle effects of EO's just be practicing this simple yet effective technique.

'Pupil Tonus' Response Testing

Another way to test EO's is the 'Pupil Tonus' approach, wherein a person uses an individual's pupils to ascertain the effect of an EO on the autonomic nervous system. This is especially effective when a person is in a state of hypnosis or trance. The person doing the pupil tonus response testing has an individual sit down and guides them through one complete cycle of the breath. The tester has the person breath in deeply, hold the breath for a few seconds, and then slowly exhale, holding the breath again for a few seconds. After this breath have the person return to their normal breathing pattern. Then, while closely watching their pupils have them smell an EO.

Does the pupil dilate or contract? If it dilates the response is parasympathetic, if it contracts the response is sympathetic. This particular response testing is actually much more detailed than I could even give here, but as a basic assessment for determining sympathetic or parasympathetic response what I've described here will suffice.

The 'Four Physio-Emotional Basics' of solar plexus response testing, which is primarily utilized by the individual themselves, and the 'Rudimentary Pulse Diagnoses' or 'Pupil Tonus' approach, which are done by a health consultant/professional, are each very effective means of ascertaining what oils to use or not use or what the overall effect upon the autonomic nervous system will be. When these tools are effectively mastered and used together they become a formidable approach to ascertaining the most effective EO's to use and the most effective means of using them.

The Biology of the Skin

One final thing concerning the biology of EO's as they effect the body is that dealing with the skin. Since most EO's are used topically (applied to the skin and surface exposed membranes) there are some general rules to remember.

Because of their extremely small molecular size EO's are generally highly absorbed into the skin. Margurite Maury, one of France's most eminent aromatherapists, used EO's on a topically exclusive basis. She seldom ever cut the EO's with fixed oils, but used the Neat preparations very sparingly (See chapter four for more information on cut versus Neat oils.) The results from her work are legendary.

As will be discussed in chapter four, contrary to popular opinion, fixed food grade oils, as a general rule, do not penetrate into the skin unless they have been specially prepared to be water miscible, which is known as a "bio-genic preparation" in the industry. This is an extensive proprietary process known only to a few cosmetic companies in the world and they hold the secrets for doing so "very-close-to-the-vest." Some fixed oils such as cold pressed hemp and grape seed oils may appear to have a very limited penetrating value when heated by vigorous massaging action upon the skin. The jury is still out on this one. As a general rule the average person will only have access to regular, food quality, fixed oils. Their uses, advantages and disadvantages are also discussed in chapter four.

As for using EO's in bath water for their therapeutic effect (which I highly recommend) its important to understand how the skin operates when placed in water.

The skin has millions of pores that open and close, depending on the environment, emotional situation and the state of the autonomic nervous system. When that bath water is drawn, either for yourself, a child or for a baby, when the body first settles into the water there is an immediate autonomic reflex to close the skin's pores. It's a spontaneous reflex humans are born with and remains with them throughout their lives.

As the body's autonomic nervous system relaxes and switches from sympathetic to parasympathetic the skin itself begins to relax and the pores then open up. On the average this takes about ten minutes. Once fully relaxed and settled the pores open wide up and for the next ten to twenty minutes the pores expel waste (as when sweating if the water is hot enough) while absorbing any components that may be in the water, such as EO's, Epsom salts, etc. At the end of the ten to twenty minutes that the skin's pores have been wide open they begin to close up again. This is another survival reflex built into humans. They close up so the body will not get too water logged and depleted of mineral electrolytes from the expelling of too much body waste.

When taking a bath with EO's remember to allow at least 20 minutes so the skin pores can cycle through their opening and closing to get the full therapeutic benefit of the EO's. Oh, one final note on essential oil baths. Pat dry the body with a towel. Don't rub yourself dry as this will pull any of the residual oils off of and out of the pores that are left from the bath.

Chapter Three

The Art of Aromatherapy

While there is a growing body of scientific research on EO's, the practical application of aromatherapy remains, by and large, an art. You would be amazed how many times individuals and companies have wasted valuable funds and time attempting to formulate aromatherapy products only to have their products fall "flat" in the marketplace. They simply don't work or people don't like them. Why is this so?

The answer is simple. There is science utilized in the identifying, harvesting and readying of the plants used for distillation. There is also science used in the engineering of the equipment used for the distillation process and in the actual distillation[6] process itself.

---

[6] This transition from science to art actually happens in the distillition process. Even though the equipment, with all its gauges and monitors, is a byproduct of science and the rules of science apply in its operation the 'art' of distillation enters in as an integral part of this process. The temperature outside relative to the inside of the facility, barometric pressure, amount of ambient humidity, season of the year and even the moon phases subtly affect the outcome of the distillation process, especially where triple distillation is concerned. Some of these factors are so subtle, albeit very real, that gauges and monitors don't pick up these anomalies that can determine if the end product is consistent from batch to batch. Only the human intuitive element that has been honed over years of distillation experience can do this on the consistent level that our industry requires. The distilling of fine single malt scotch whiskey is somewhat similar to the distilling of EO's. Over two centuries of distilling fine single malt whiskey has shown that the more the human element (the 'art') is incorporated into making these whiskey's the higher their quality. The most reputable

However, once the oils have been prepared, the process of blending those oils into usable consumer products is an art, therefore science must now take the back seat previously held by the art.

It's a sort of like a 'Spontaneous Fire Drill' (previously called a Chinese Fire Drill) where the art (that has been sitting in the passenger seat) and science (which has been in the driver's seat) suddenly switch seats at a stop light. Now science must take the passenger seat, while art takes the drivers position. In the field of aromatherapy, like music, dance, painting or any other creative act that appeals to our senses, there is a subjective intuition needed that technical know how can never replace.

This is because artistic thinking is holistic thinking whereas science is fractured or reductionistic thinking. It can only look at the pieces, not the whole. This is why the scientific mind alone can't quite grasp the holistic concepts found in aromatherapy (or herbalism for that matter).

The American scientific community, especially the medico-pharmaceutical side, has a propensity for not accepting anything outside of its own community, even when they know little or nothing about the subject at hand. No where is this more obvious than in the area of aromatherapy.

---

internationally known distillery houses of aromatic essential oils know this and apply the human factor heavily in their operations, and it shows in the consistent quality of their EO's.

The Europeans – A Holistic Approach

In Europe, the leading continent in the world on aromatherapy and EO's research, they have learned (and honored) the time proven holistic principle of the Spontaneous Fire Drill where the science and art of aromatherapy are concerned. In their industry they use science to make the actual EO's, research their biological effects and so forth. However, when it comes time for compounding, blending and formulating the consumer based products, the scientists yield to those with the artistic knack. Since machines and analytical devices don't have noses, tongues and a nervous system that responds with phsyiological and emotional changes, it takes a human being to judge the probable response of other human beings to a given aromatic product.

The culinary arts of France, Italy, Switzerland and Spain rely heavily on aromatic spices and herbs, the same spices and herbs EO's are distilled from. In the bakery trade of these nations they rely heavily on complex flavoring blends that are EO based and blended in the artful fashion I've described. I might here say that the master chefs of these countries only use all natural ingredients in their cooking, including the EO based flavorings.

Even the medicinal use of EO's in Europe is heavily influenced by the artful aspect of the blenders skill. This skill depends not only on the scientifically understood characteristics of the EO's, but on the artistic expression utilized in the final formulating of a blend for a specific individual or situation at hand.

In fact, if you want to learn to be effective in using aromatherapy you need to train your own nose and taste. You must learn to blend EO's with an artistic sense, using your nose and tongue to judge the result, just like a person who takes up brushes and oils to create a fine masterpiece assesses his work with his eyes. Folks, no matter how you look at it the practical applications of aromatherapy is an art!

A Question of Quality

Many of you reading this book are consumers or purveyors of herbal products. Have you noted that the less expensive the herbal product is the more inconsistent the results? I recall my own recent experience with three herbal products that were being sold by a wholesale shopping club I belong to. They were ginkgo, St. John's Wort and echinacea. Imagine, 60 caplet bottles at 1/3 the price of other brands I had been buying. So I bought some of each. They were definitely inferior products, since I didn't get the anticipated results I had gotten from the quality brands I paid more for.

Perhaps the herbs had been processed to adversely affect their efficacy. It is possible they weren't even the herbal species I thought I was buying. Adulteration and substitution of one plant for another is common in the herb industry. In fact, I later learned that my suspicions were confirmed by consumer research groups and a couple of reputable companies own analysis of these products.

The bottom line is "Cheap is Cheap" and only makes for cheap results. Essential oils are the same, only more so. The less expensive (which means they are either synthetic or poor distillates) the cheaper the results. In this case, however, poor quality EO's may not only be ineffective, they may also cause bad reactions and dangerous effects.

Europe has gone light years ahead in this aspect while here in America there is still a prevailing tendency to want to synthesize anything and everything. We want things to be scientifically synthesized in cheap assembly line fashion. What Americans don't realize, but the Europeans learned long ago, is that the cheaper something is, the less effective its results will be.

I can't name how many times someone brings me an EO product from the store shelf or some marketing company and I cringe when I investigate the product. Having an excellent nose, which I have carefully trained for blending aromatherapy products, and an even keener sense of taste, I am able to very accurately judge the quality of EO-based products.

Recently I was introduced to a large herbal company's foray into the aromatherapy market. One of their distributors showed me a lavender oil they had been using for a few years and the lavender oil this company was introducing through their distribution network. The person was convinced that the new lavender oil product was of poorer quality than the lavender product she had used all these years. I then took both of the products and put them through a simple test right there on the spot. The product she had previously been using was a good product, but it was slightly more resinous and cottony in its effect upon my nose. On the other hand, the new label was brighter and more airy and seemed to have a depth the other didn't possess.

What amazed this individual was when I had her take a slow sustained breath of each (clearing her nose between the two) she found that she could actually smell a subtle 'fresh' lavender blossom smell that would creep through periodically while she inhaled it. The upshot being that the new lavender product was definitely of a much higher quality while the older product she had used was somewhat inferior.

It further amazed her when she came back and talked to me two hours later. We found that the old lavender product's aroma had almost completely disappeared, while the new lavender was still full and complete, having only lost a small amount of it top notes, as any high grade aromatic EO would do. What had I done that was so different from what she was doing to detect quality?

My criteria for determining the quality of an EO is not simply inhaling an EO while it remains in the bottle. This is an important part but only one part of establishing quality. After inhaling an EO in the bottle I next take a drop of each oil and put it on the heel (or the wrist) of each separate hand and again inhale each. Now we are going to start smelling a pattern emerge between the two. One is going to begin to stand out from the other. From there I then vigorously rub each into the skin to create enough warmth that will release the components of the EO. Each hand where the oil has been rubbed into the skin is then slowly and deeply inhaled, allowing for a break between each hand. From this a rudimentary and fairly accurate conclusion of EO quality can be ascertained. It takes practice and an understanding of the oils being dealt with, but I have never had this technique fail me.

My neurological makeup is also quite consistent, and therefore makes me a good neuro-responsive tester (as I described in the 'Four Physio-Emotional Basics' of solar plexus response testing). A person doesn't need to tell me what an EO product was blended for, just let me get into 'my space' and try it, and I'll tell you what it's doing to the body. This includes both physiological and emotional responses. The blender's art takes years of practice to acquire and can never be rushed.

I generally find that if a company places a large emphasis on quality control and consistency of its products, they usually carry that same protocol through to the development of a line of essential oil products. Some stumble along due to their over scientificizing, but even they eventually get the picture and call on the art of a qualified experienced aromatherapy blender to get the job done right. Look for these kinds of companies to do business with, because it's so easy to get ripped off and not even know its happening to you.

To help you find high quality aromatic essential oils I have established the following set of rules. Look for oils that can meet these standards and you can be assured of the highest quality products.

Criteria & Standards for Selecting EO's.

a. EO's should be unadulterated, 100% pure and derived from botanical (plant) materials, not synethesized.

b. EO's should be distilled at the highest quality level available. Many of the best, such as lavender, bergamot and chamomile, are triple distilled and often carry the 'fine' or 'extra' designation.

c. EO's should be analyzed and tested to be the highest quality available—which includes being free of pesticide and herbicide residues.

d. EO's should be fresh, meaning the product inventory should be properly rotated (oldest product sold first) and the products should be appropriately packaged, sealed, and batch numbered for quality assurance.

e. EO's should be sourced from the areas of the world where the highest quality of oil can be obtained for a particular plant. Suggestions for best sources for various oils are found in chapter four.

f. EO's should be packaged in easy-to-use containers which enable controlled dispensing to reduce or eliminate mess and waste.

g. EO's should be competively priced in accordance to the quality of oil being offered.

h. EO's should be properly labeled, meaning the product contains exactly what is on the label.

i. EO formulas should be developed only by experienced EO blenders who have developed the art of combining oils through practice and clinicial experience.

j. EO's should be certified organic when organic plant material is available.

As you can see, I've put together quite a list of criteria for you. Pay careful attention to it. Years of clinical application and blending experience have taught me a lot, particularly in the area of quality control (or the lack of it). I've worked directly with some of the largest EO manufacturers and wholesalers to learn these principles.

I've dealt with some real quality operations at the manufacturing level who once they understood what I required always came through for me. It's the wholesalers and distributor based operations you have to watch out for.

Lower grade EO's (rejected for USP and/or fine custom perfume usage) are often sold on the secondary market as Fine grade products. Even worse is the improperly distilled oils that are clouded (at room temperature), have sediment or strong stratification of the constituents. These are not fit for human use of any kind. I'm even aware of instances where improperly distilled EO's were put through a filtration process to remove the clouding and sediment to make them appear a quality product.

Making Sense of Product Labels

Earlier in this work I discussed the subjective nature of aromatherapy. This is part of the reason aromatherapy is an art. As part of the art and for the benefit of the consumer at large I am calling upon the companies that manufacture and market EO based products to dispense with the prevailing labeling scheme that makes arbitrary claims for specific emotional effects and responses. Claiming that a product will have a specific emotional response is confusing to the consumer. For instance, I am aware of one product that is called 'concentrate.' That product happens to make me feel more alert. An alert state can often distract one from a task at hand and hence diminish their powers of concentration.

What is labeled as being a meditative blend too often makes a person feel agitated and flighty, definitely not meditative feelings. Likewise, something labeled as invigorating often has the effect of making a person feel foggy, sluggish and disoriented. Labeling schemes need to be more abstract, but at the same time accurate, leaving the decision of what to use for which on a more objective level.

There are effective means of ascertaining which blend is best for a person at a given time. Smell and/or Taste Response Testing and how it effects the solar plexus response, Rudimentary Pulse Diagnoses and/or Pupil Tonus Response Testing are all good methods. These testing methods were discussed in the previous chapter.

'Neat' and 'Cut'

EO's come in two forms—Neat and Cut. Neat means that the EO's are in a pure unadulterated state—100 percent pure essential oil. Cut means that another carrier agent or dilutant has been used. Common carrier agents for EO's include water, honey, vinegars & wines, fats, alcohol, mineral oil, glycol, waxes and vegetable oils. Cutting a Neat EO is usually done for application purposes, such as massage oils or unguents. It may also be done to aid in localized applications, such as ear or nose drops.

As far as the natural holistic applications of EO's are concerned, alcohol, mineral oil and glycol are unacceptable means of cutting Neat EO's. Honey is one of the best ways of presenting EO's for internal nutritional therapy use. Vegetable oils can also be used similar to honey, but is best used to Cut EO's for topical therapeutic purposes.

Glycols?

Glycol is used extensively in the foods industry (artificial vanilla, artificial lemon and orange flavoring, etc.) and is a component that is the second to last step in the final manufacturing of automotive anti-freeze.[7] Many people have a high sensitivity to

---

[7] Cheap "border town" Mexican vanillan (artificial vanilla) flavoring is actually made with automotive anti-freeze – hence

glycol (especially the skin) and in some people with weak liver activity or exhausted liver activity there is a cumulative effect when glycol is used (internally) over long periods of time.

Mineral oil?

Mineral oil is the most widely used base in body work oils and lotions that use EO's in the industry. It is a cheap agent derived from petroleum and is a good holder of EO's. Therein lies one of the problems of mineral oil. Because it does not absorb into the skin or through tissues it's tight holding onto the EO's does not allow for transfer and absorption into the body. Thus, the benefits of the EO's are largely lost.

Mineral oil also clogs the pores of the skin and prevents the skin from breathing and releasing metabolic toxins. Contrary to popular belief, mineral oil does not moisturize the skin, in fact it contributes to the drying and roughening of skin. Mineral oil should never, except in extreme emergency situations, be considered an option in aromatherapy.

Alcohol?

Alcohol is used in herbal tinctures and toiletries (i.e. perfumes, aftershaves, colognes, etc.). It is also used in liniments due to its surface cooling action. Alcohol is a good solvent for extracting the aromatic constituents of a plant and allows for a complete

---

the FDA warnings and ban on importation of most Mexican companies manufacturing flavoring agents.

diffusion of EO's into the medium. It also allows the camphorous and menthol components to maintain their overall effect. However, alcohol renders the other therapeutic actions of EO's and EO blends completely inert. This is because the alcohol breaks up many of the components of an EO, which in essence (no pun intended) alters its therapeutic applications and changes the oil into something unnatural. Even liniments have been proven to have limited therapeutic value beyond the massaging associated with their use and the cooling effect of the alcohol.

Water!

Water is the least effective carrier of EO's, but it does have some limited use. When used as a foot bath or full bath, water, especially with Epsom salts, is a surface dispersant of EO's enabling the EO's to drape about the body. Especially as one gets out of the tub and stands for a few moments to allow the EO's to penetrate into the skin pores. A couple of drops of EO's in a glass of water is also very good, especially in lemon, clove or lavender oil, because each have a strong disinfecting action on the water.

Honey!

Honey not only acts as a very effective carrier of EO's into the mouth and down into the digestive system, it holds onto the EO's until well down the throat and honey itself has an antiseptic action that compliments EO's. In a pinch, when no other carriers or cutting agents are available honey can be used to dress a wound or soothe the skin. The usual mix for topical use is 1 part EO to nine parts honey.

Vinegars & Wines!

Vinegars and wines are not a whole lot better than water as carriers except that they have distinct therapeutic effects themselves. Used topically they are cooling and toning to the skin. Internally, vinegar is disinfecting and antibacterial to the stomach. Wine is an excellent replenisher of essential mineral electrolytes, it mildly stimulates digestive actions while relaxing the digestive system itself. The low amount of alcohol has little immediate effect on an EO's therapeutic outcome due to the short duration the EO is left to soak in a glass of wine. It is best used with EO's as a digestive tonic and mild appetite stimulant.

Fats!

Today fats, especially plant source fats, are typically used in the cosmetics industry as bases for making perfume "absolute." The word absolute means that it is solid at room temperature. Absolutes are one of the best ways to preserve an EO almost indefinitely. The tombs of ancient Egypt had urns that still contained unguents (rudimentary absolutes) with enough of the EO's still intact to know by smell what they were – 4,000 years later!

Waxes!

Paraffin wax, derived from petroleum, is used in cheap common lotions. Actually paraffin wax is just the solid counterpart to mineral oil. Petroleum jelly (Vaseline), another petroleum product that is a sort of hybridized mineral oil and paraffin wax combination falls into the same category. I do not recommend the use of paraffin wax and only in the most extreme emergency would use petroleum jelly when no beeswax, honey or other fixed oils was available.

Beeswax is one of the best of all waxes to use. It is found in the best natural salves, ointments and wax based unguents there is. It is friendly to EO's, it readily mixes with and micro-encapsulates the EO's molecules and does not rancify or degrade with time.

Fixed Oils!

EO's are classified as 'Aromatic' oils, meaning they evaporate, are flammable to one degree or another, and they do not stain cloth. Vegetable oils are classified as 'Fixed' oils, meaning they do not evaporate, are not flammable, and will permanently stain cloth. Fixed oils act as 'Fixatives' when used to cut EO's, meaning they have the property of keeping the aromatic oil from evaporating. They also reduce the flammability index of EO's.

Vegetable oils are generally the preferred means of cutting Neat EO's. They allow strong EO's to be easily diluted to an appropriate strength. They can also help to extend expensive oils. I've found that the fixed oils of Olive and Almond (sweet) are two of the best, but because of their high viscosity (thickness) they often need to be cut themselves with a lighter oil, such as safflower, sesame, peanut or grape seed oil. I prefer grape seed oil, because of its relatively reasonable cost and light aroma that compliments the aroma of other EO's. I often use Almond oil cut with an appropriate amount of grape seed oil to produce a likeable consistency. This is a good combination for most general purposes.

However, when dealing with some tough therapeutic situations, cold pressed hemp oil appears to be even better. There is strong evidence that cold pressed hemp oil may be one of the most therapeutically enhancing fixed oil's there is. It has been used for food and therapy purposes long before the white man even set food on this hemisphere. Thus, it has stood the test of time. It is the highest oil in essential fatty acids known, even better than flaxseed oil.

Along with its own therapeutic action, hemp is extremely friendly to EO's, it is very stable and has a high degree of emollient (softening and lubricating) activity. Because of hemp's ability to break down into smaller molecular chains when worked over (i.e. being vigorously massaged against the skin), there are indications that some limited penetration into body tissues may ensue, which means it may be one of the best carriers of EO's into the skin. The jury is still out on this one.

Hemp oil was at one time the most widely used, all-purpose oil for food, cosmetic, mechanical and therapeutic purposes in America. Then, the petrochemical industry introduced mineral oil (and all its quackish "cure-all" derivations) in the late 19th and early 20th century. They also prevailed on the United States government to outlaw the agricultural production of hemp. Today, due to overwhelming scientific and medical evidence and relaxed legal regulations they allow agricultural production and non-medical use of hemp, hemp oil is enjoying a renewed revival in the foods, cosmetics and health industry.

The Skin Penetration Myth of Fixed Oils

It should be remembered that fixed oils, in and of themselves, have no real penetration into the skin. This belief is a myth that has long been disproved. Even hemp oil, if it does have limited penetration, cannot do so until the oil is "worked over" or rubbed to break it down. This means that to simply apply a fixed oil that contains EO's to the skin and lightly spread it will have very little therapeutic effect except in the most extreme cases of wasting. The oil must be kneaded and worked upon the skin so as to heat up the surface of the skin. As the oils come into active contact with the heated skin the therapeutic value of the EO's is released from the fixed oil and absorbed into the skin. All massage therapists and body workers know the importance of this. This applies to soft temple massages for headaches, scalp massage for tension, a stripping massage of the neck and shoulders, etc.

One note of warning—never use a fixed oil to cut EO's for use in an aromatherapy diffuser. It won't

work. The fixed oil is too thick and viscous and will
only gum up the diffuser.

Chapter Four

The Practice of Aromatherapy

The use of EO's as therapeutic holistic adjuncts to herbalism, nutritional counseling, body work, ortho-molecular psychology and hypnotherapy (and all its derivations) is experiencing a huge rise in popularity. Not only is the health practitioner aware of this, the consumer at large is tuned in to the value of EO's. The demand for EO products has skyrocketed in the past decade alone, and the growth potential will continue well into the next decade. It is due to the increased demand and decreased supply that quality control and formulations done by experienced qualified blenders of EO's products will become more important than ever.

In this chapter, I will address the basic therapeutic uses of single EO's as well as some sample blends for specific purposes. First, however, we will look at the single EO's. Here are some of the characteristics and information we will be reviewing for each of them.

Cooling EO's and Warming EO's

First, I've classified EO's into two basic categories, warming and cooling. This is similar to the Oriental natural philosophy expressed in the concept of Yin and Yang.

A cooling EO tends to have a settling effect on the body, in the extreme it would even be sedating. A warming EO tends to have an enlivening effect on the body, which taken in the extreme would be agitating.

Some EO's are so "middle of the road" that it's difficult to ascertain if they are cooling or warming. Here again we utilize the principle of dominance, meaning we ascertain if there is more of a cooling or warming dominance and categorize it accordingly.

The Cooling Aromatic EO's

Bergamot (Citrus bergamia)

Chamomile, Roman (Chamaemelum nobile)

Citronella (Cymbopogon nardus)

Coriander (Coriandrum sativum)

Fennel seed (Foeniculum vulgare)

Geranium (Pelargonium graveolens)

Grapefruit, Pink (Citrus paradisi)

Lavender (Lavendula officinalis)

Lemon (Citrus limonum)

Lemongrass (Cymbopogon citratus)

Marjoram (Origanum majorana)

Nutmeg (Myristica fragrans)

Patchouli (Pogostemon patchouli)

Rose Moroc Clear (Rosa variety)

Sandalwood (Santalum album)

Ylang Ylang Extra (Canaga odorata)

The Warming Aromatics EO's

Cajeput (Melaleuca leucadendron)

Cardamom (Elettaria cardamomum)

Cinnamon (Cinnamonum zeylanicum)

Clary Sage (Salva sclarea)

Clove (Eugenia caryophyllata)

Eucalyptus (Eucalyptus globulus)

Garlic (Allium sativum)

Ginger (Zingiber officinale)

Juniper (Juniperus communis)

Pine (Pinus sylvestris)

Peppermint (Mentha piperita)

Rosemary (Rosmarinus officinalis)

Tea Tree (Maleleuca alternifolia)

Thyme, Red (Thymus vulgaris)

Best Source & Plant Part

Over my years of research in aromatherapy, I have determined the areas of the world where the finest quality EO's are derived. I have made note of this in this book along with which plant parts should be used to distill the highest quality oils. Good grades of oils may be had from other sources, but the sources listed in this book are where one finds the highest grade.

Aroma

I have described the qualities of aroma each oil possesses. This is based on the overall quality the oil exhibits. I have attempted to keep a description of these qualities as generic as possible. For instance, when I use the term 'citrus' most everyone generally acknowledges what that means. There is a fairly widespread consensus on the meaning of citrus. The same is true of the other words used to describe the overall aromatic quality of an oil.

Usage

All of the uses described in this chapter refer to uses of the oils for either topical application or inhalation. Although EO's may also be used internally for therapeutic purposes, the clinical applications of EO's for internal use requires extensive clinical therapeutic experience. In fact, unless you have very precise knowledge of the oils, DO NOT USE EO's INTERNALLY. I mention any internal therapeutic use for professional purposes only. Because they are so potent, they can easily be misused and are in many cases toxic when ingested. Therefore, except where noted otherwise, all uses of EO's mentioned in this text are associated with topical application and inhalation.

For each oil I have listed it's healing properties and specific uses. I have also indicated its typical neuro-emotional effects and usage. However, keep in mind that the neuro-emotional effects are very subjective (as discussed in Chapter 2) and that some individuals will react differently to various oils depending on the conditioned responses of their nervous system.

Contraindications

Remember that you are using the essence of a plant, the part of the plant that carries the signature of all that it is, in its most potent form. On the alchemical wheel of life (air, water, fire and earth) EO's represent the element of fire. So, it is essential that no one gets 'burned' from their misuse. Contraindications are the symptoms and conditions for which an EO should be avoided. Please pay careful attention to these cautions and warnings when choosing oils for therapeutic purposes.

Index to the Oils

The following pages contain an index to various essential oils and their uses:

Bergamot (*Citrus bergamia*)

Classification: Cooling.

Plant Part(s): Fruit rind.

Best Source: Italy.

Aroma: Medium, sweet, freshening, biting citrus, and fruity.

General Usage:

Anti-Depressant (Mild)	Digestive Aid
Antiparasitic	Fever Reducing
Appetite Stimulant	Soothes Muscles

Specific Topical Usage:

Blemished (bleached) skin	Eczema
	Sores
Burns (light)	Varicose veins

It is also used in Europe as a suntan oil (mixed with aloe vera especially).

Neuro-emotional Usage:

Confusion	Feeling "Old"
Depression	Feeling Emotionally "Bloated"
Feeling "Lopsided"	

Emotional Effect: Helps a person feel happy, cheerful and "clean."

Contraindications: Chills, overeating, flaccid muscles, headaches (vaso-dilative —throbbing or pounding headaches), compulsive behavior, overly mental individuals, and hurried or rushed feelings.

General Information:

Bergamot is a major component in many citrus or spice based toiletries. The best quality comes from the Mediterranean coastal regions of Italy, which provides the world's supply of premium quality bergamot.

As a febrifuge (fever reducer) I recommend the following regime. Add lavender (1 drop) and bergamot (1 drop) to a teaspoon of glycerin and swallow slowly. Fifteen minutes later serve a tepid tea of elder flowers and peppermint or a tepid tea of yarrow flowers and peppermint. Do this regime every two hours until the fever breaks. It's especially effective on children.

For sore muscles, place a couple of drops on the shoulders and then rub in vigorously. This helps to alleviate muscle tension.

For a wonderful cooling effect on an overwhelmed mind rub one to two drops of bergamot into the palms of the hand and then place the cupped hands over the mouth and nose while breathing. Bergamot is mildly relaxing to the senses but when used in excess can have the effect of throwing the neuro-emotional state into malaise. It is best indicated for intermittent depression where vision problems seem to persist.

Cajeput (*Melaleuca leucadendron*)

Classification: Warming.

Best Source: Australia.

Plant Part(s): Leaves.

Aroma: Light, eucalyptus-like, very "herby (musty medicinal aroma)."

General Usage:

Antifungal

Digestive Spasms

Earache

Intestinal Parasites

Laryngitis

Nervous Vomiting

Respiratory Problems

Rheumatic Neuralgia

Skin and Wound Healing (with little or no scaring)

Skin Irritations

Toothache

Specific Topical Usage:

Alopecia

Balding Scalp Care

Skin Inflammations

Neuro-emotional Usage:

"Creepy-Crawling" Sensations

Apathetic

Crabby

Cranky

Enervated

Feeling "Bugged," Edgy

Irritated

Emotional Effect: Awakening and stimulating.

Contraindications: Atonic digestion, general malaise and emotional flaccidity.

General Information:

Cajeput is initially cooling then turns warming through an expansive diffusive action. This is why cajeput is one of the best EO's for earaches. Cajeput (1 part) and lavender (1 part) are two of the oldest European blends for ear problems. It is also used in conjunction with garlic oil (2 parts cajeput, 2 parts lavender and 1 part garlic) for ear problems. When used in the ears these oils should be cut with olive oil so that the EO's represent only 7 percent of the finished oil. Two to four drops of this cut mixture is then placed in the ear. (Do not use uncut or undiluted oils in the ear.)

I have used this blend with excellent results for blocked ear tubes and earaches. I have also applied it to the back of the throat (4 drops) for thrush on small children. It's strong and they may fuss for a moment, but that soon passes as the effects set in.

Cardamom (*Elettaria cardamomum*)

Classification: Warming.

Best Source: India.

Plant Part(s): Seeds.

Aroma: Heavy, sweetish, spicy, lightly blossomy, and balsamic (soft warming resinoid character).

General Usage:

Carminative (Expels Gas)

Cold (Sluggish) And Dry Reproductive System

Digestive Tonic

Diuretic

Loss of Appetite

Nausea

Vaso-Constrictive (Tension) Headaches

Specific Topical Usage: None.

Neuro-emotional Usage:

Confusion

Feelings of Being Heavy-Headed

For Cold And Distant Feelings

Mental Chatter

Mental Fatigue

Repressed Sexual Feelings

Timidity

Unsociable

Urge To "Hide-In-A-Cave"

Emotional Effect: Uplifting, mentally clarifying, expressive.

Contraindications: Overly stimulated metabolism. Overly sexed libido.

General Information:

Cardamom is referred to as a 'forbidden seed' in the ancient sacred texts of Hinduism. It is warming to the system with a special affinity to the pelvic regions of the body. In the Tibetan plateau cardamom seed is the primary spice in their butter tea that is a national drink known for its warming effect on the body. From a scientific point of view the cardamom cuts the negative aspects of the high butter content as well as contributing to the warming effect of the overall tea. It is excellent for reducing flatulence caused by undigested starchy foods.

Chamomile, Roman
(*Chamaemelum nobile*)

Classification: Cooling.

Best Source: Hungary or Egypt.

Plant Part(s): Flowers.

Aroma: Medium, sweet, herby, and strongly present.

General Usage:

Antiinflammatory

Antiseptic

Antispasmodic

Astringent

Burns

Cicatrizing (Skin Cell Regenerating)

Eyelid Problems

Herpes

Overly Oily Skin

Specific Topical Usage:

Acne

Disinfect Purulent (Oozing Slow Healing) Wounds

Exfoliation (Accelerate)

General Skin Care

Skin Inflammation

Sunburn

Neuro-emotional Usage:

Feeling "Rough-On-The-Edges"

Grasping

Hysteria

Insomnia

Intermittent Nervous Depression

Neurotic Episodes

Obsessive Behavior   Uptight

Emotional Effect: Calming, settling and soothing.

Contraindications: Should not be used where there is prolonged exposure to direct sunlight. Also contraindicated in chronic anxiety and narcolepsy.

General Information:

Chamomile, long known for its digestive qualities, is also used extensively in aesthetician skin care products (especially in Europe) due to its antiseptic and skin regenerative qualities. A skin and wound healing blend can be made that consists of lavender (3 parts) and chamomile (1 part). Chamomile has long been used as a natural bleaching aid to blonde hair and to lighten skin. Chamomile EO is extremely potent, containing the richest amount of azulene of any EO. The azulene, which gives chamomile oil its dark blue color, is the active constituent known for its benefit to skin and mucous tissues. Like lavender, chamomile has a cicatrizing action upon the skin. This means it is able to accelerate healing processes that result in less discomfort and reduced scarring.

Cinnamon (*Cinnamonum zeylanicum*)

Classification: Warming.

Best Source: Ceylon (Sri Lanka).

Plant Part(s): Bark.

Aroma: Medium clove-like, spicy-sweet, and warm.

General Usage:

Anti-Fungal

Anti-hemorrhagic

Bites and Stings

Debility (Particularly Flu)

Digestive Problems

Flatulence

Mildly Aphrodisiac

Reduces Spasms in the Gastro-Intestinal Tract

Stimulates Starch Digestion

Specific Topical Usage:

Lifeless and Sallow Skin

Skin Parasites.

Neuro-emotional Usage:

Fears and Concerns

Feeling "All Bound Up"

Feeling Choked

Frigidity

High Anxiety

Hysteria

Melancholic Feelings with a Sense of Fragility

Emotional Effect: Helps a person feel warm and safe.

Contraindications: Not for use with overly active digestion (acidic indigestion).

General Information:

Cinnamon is derived from the bark of the cinnamon tree. It is especially good for debilitating conditions when 1 to 2 drops of cinnamon is mixed with a slippery elm gruel. This combination is seldom refused by a weak digestive system. Cinnamon (1 part) used with lavender (1 part) is one of the best surface antidotes to poisonous bites and stings there is. It will often stave off any wasting of tissue if used expediently. It is an excellent anti-haemorrhagic especially when used with capsicum, and the two together will encourage an anti-shock response.

Citronella (*Cymbopogon nardus*)

Classification: Cooling.

Best Source: Madagascar.

Plant Part(s): Grass.

Aroma: Light but penetrating, wet hay, and amber-like.

General Usage:

Disinfectant (Mild)

Household Cleaner Refresher

Insect Repellant

Lice and Skin Parasites

Rheumatism

Specific Topical Usage:

Insect Repellant

Skin Anti-Parasitic

Neuro-emotional Usage:

Mental Fogginess

Sluggish Emotions

Emotional Effect: Clarifies and refreshes (when used sparingly)

Contraindications: *Use sparingly. Do not use internally.* Should not be used on individuals prone to enervation. People who suffer from headaches or migraines of all kinds should not use citronella.

General Information:

Citronella has fallen into disrepute in the last 20 years due to its being one of the most commonly used essences worldwide in soap making and household cleaner manufacturing, and its being the main aromatic component in EO adulterants. In deed, notoriety and commonality has taken its toll. I personally consider Citronella to be a necessary part of a user friendly aromatherapy program. In fact, next to eucalyptus, citronella may be the most user friendly of EO's. An excellent all natural aromatic insect repellant can be made by taking geranium (1 part) and citronella (4 parts) and cutting the Neat blend with a non-scented lotion (EO blend being 10 to 20 percent of finished lotion). This EO's insect repellant blend also works great on cats and dogs (just don't put on the eyes or nose of the animal).

Clary Sage (*Salva sclarea*)

Classification: Warming.

Best Source: France.

Plant Part(s): Herb.

Aroma: Light, smoke ash, hay like, and sweet.

General Usage:

Anti-inflammatory	Bronchitis
Anti-Spasmodic	

Specific Topical Usage:

General Hair Care	Inflamed Skin Conditions
General Skin Care	
Hair Loss	

Neuro-emotional Usage:

Agitated	Feeling "Rough on the Edges"
Be-Moaning Everything	Uninspired
Depression	

Emotional Effect: Blissful and euphoric.

Contraindications: High anxiety.

General Information:

Clary sage is the most aromatically therapeutic of all sages. Unlike sage dalmation, clary sage's aroma exhibits a decidedly 'smokey' character. I believe that this EO has a similar physiological effect upon the respiratory system as a fumigant (smudges or therapeutic incenses) does. The smokey character of the aroma seems to indicate this and the overall therapeutic action on the bronchials bears this out. A drop of clary sage on a mosquito bite with applied pressure by the thumbnail will almost always clear up the irritation.

Clove (*Eugenia caryophyllata*)

Classification: Warming.

Best Source: Madagascar.

Plant Part(s): Flower buds.

Aroma: Heavy, spicy, biting, sweet, and warm.

General Usage:

Anti-Parasitic

Antiseptic (3 To 4 Times Greater Than Phenol)

Antispasmodic

Insect Repellant

Topical Oral Pain Relief (Anodyne)

Specific Topical Usage:

Calluses

Insect Bites

Purulent Wounds

Skin Parasites

Skin Ulcers

Warts (Specific For)

Neuro-emotional Usage:

Denial

Incoherent

Mental Fatigue

Post-Traumatic Shock

Emotional Effect: Present and aware.
Special Note: Clove should be used with extreme caution on the skin, since many people (especially Caucasians) exhibit more of a topical sensitivity to this oil than many other oils. Use with care.

The Practice of Aromatherapy

Contraindications: Not to be used during pregnancy. Skin allergy problems. Obsessive/compulsive behavior (clove seems to drive it).

General Information:

Clove is one of the most powerful antiseptic agents known. It is also one of the most researched. An effective user-friendly home based antiseptic formula consists of a "Bronner's™" type soap to which 1 percent clove is added. This will make the best antiseptic handwash there is. For a household cleaning formula mix a "Simple Green™" type of cleaner as per instructions and to the ready-to-use cleaner add 1/2 to 1 percent clove oil, depending on the cleaning job. To give the household cleaner a "Pinesol™" character add .10 to .20 percent Pine oil (which is disinfecting as well).

Coriander (*Coriandrum sativum*)

Classification: Cooling.

Best Source: Russia.

Plant Part(s): Seed.

Aroma: Ethereal lightness, aromatic, and fruity.

General Usage:

Aphrodisiac

Flatulence

Gaseous Digestion

Gastrointestinal
Spasms

Loss of Appetite

Rheumatic Pains

Swallowing Air

Specific Topical Usage: None.

Neuro-emotional Usage:

Emotionally Driven
Shock

"Feel-Like-Crap"

"It-Hurts-Too-Much-
To-Love"

Lack of Feeling

Loss of Memory

Mental Fatigue

Emotional Effect: Relaxes and clarifies the mind.

Contraindications: Do not use during pregnancy (has abortifacant actions) or as part of a weight loss program due to its being one of the strongest appetite stimulants known. Overly sensitized emotional feelings.

General Information:

Coriander is a sweet aromatic EO with many of the physiological benefits of Anise, only much easier on the nervous system. It is a unique digestant in that while it stimulates digestive activity, it does so in a cooling manner by not increasing hydrochloric acid production, making it an excellent starch digestive aid. A simple internal use digestive balancing aid can be made by blending cardamom (1 part), ginger (1 part), peppermint (1 part) and coriander (2 parts), and taking 2 to 4 drops with or immediately prior to a meal.

Fennel seed (*Foeniculum vulgare*)

Classification: Cooling.

Best Source: N. Italy or Central Europe.

Plant Part(s): Seed.

Aroma: Medium, like aniseed, warm-like, and very sweet.

General Usage:

Anti-Parasitic (Vermifuge)

Flatulence

Gastric Spasms

General Digestive Tonic

Insufficient Breast Milk (Glactagogue)

Laxative (Mild)

Urinary Obstructions

Weight Control Aid

Specific Topical Usage:

Cellulite (As a Neat Rub on the Specific Area)

Neuro-emotional Usage:

"In-Over-My-Head"

"The-Whole-World-On-My-Shoulders" Feeling

Bloated Feelings

Carrying A Heavy Load

Cemented Binding Feelings

Feelings Like a Dream Where You Struggle Running but Can't Move Forward

Overexcited

Overwhelmed

Emotional Effect: Calm, endearing and careful (as opposed to cynical).

Contraindications: Excessive breast milk production. Diarrhea. Underweight individuals.

General Information:

Fennel is one of the sweetest tasting EO's available. It is a soothing digestant, which contributes to its mild laxative action and anti-spasmodic activity. Even the EO has an affinity for the adrenals, which contributes to its digestive tonic action. Fennel is an excellent weight control aid because it stimulates the satiation response of the taste buds and stomach. Used in small amounts it is an excellent aid with mineral electrolyte replenishment programs. By itself fennel is an excellent glactagogue, however it moderates the powerful parasympathetic effects of lemongrass (itself a glactagogue). Blend lemongrass (1 part) and fennel (2 parts) and add to a glass of hot blessed thistle/marsh mallow tea to encourage breast milk production.

Eucalyptus (*Eucalyptus globulus*)

Classification: Warming.

Best Source: Australia or Spain.

Plant Part(s): Leaves.

Aroma: Light, penetrating, medicinal, camphoraceous, and resiny.

General Usage:

Anti-Fungal
Antiseptic
Antiviral
Blood Sugar
Cicatrizes Burns
    (Heals With A
Minimum Of
Scaring)
Congestion
Expectorant
Joint and Muscle Pain
Migraines
Respiratory Problems

Specific Topical Usage:

Antiseptic
Blisters
Cuts
Skin Cleanser
Sores
Wounds

Neuro-emotional Usage:

General Mental
    Malaise
Mentally and
    Emotionally Irritated
Trouble Concentrating

Emotional Effect: Expansive and spaceless.

Contraindications: Dry mucous membranes. Where eucalyptus sensitivity appears to be imminent.

General Information:

Eucalyptus is the most commonly used aromatic EO worldwide for everything from cough drops to emergency antiseptic wound cleaning. It can be added to boiling water to inhale for as a decongestant. Simply place a towel over the head and the head over the steaming water with the eucalyptus oil. This same arrangement of putting a few drops of eucalyptus in boiling water every few minutes is an effective way to antiseptically clean the air in an emergency. Eucalyptus is the best oil to cut all other EO's for aromatherapy diffuser use. This is due to extremely low viscosity, high diffusability and volatility index. Typically 5 to 15 percent of other EO's are cut with 85 to 95 percent eucalyptus. The exact amount depends on a combination of the viscosity and action of the EO. For example, sandalwood is 5 percent or less due to its high viscosity and extremely active aroma, whereas pine or lavender are added to the mixture at up to 15 percent due to their low viscosity and manageable aroma level. Thyme, though it has a low viscosity, has its highly active thymol components; therefore it should not exceed 7 percent of the diffuser blend.

Garlic (*Allium sativum*)

Classification: Warming.

Best Source: France.

Plant Part(s): Bud.

Aroma: Heavy, garlicky, pungent, and penetrating.

General Usage:

Antibacterial

Antibiotic

Anti-Fungal

Anti-Parasitic

Antiseptic

Antiviral

Blood Pressure

Edema (Water Retention)

Otitis (Inflammation of the Ear Canal)

Specific Topical Usage:

Abscesses

Calluses

Fungal Infections.

Insect Bites

Skin Parasites

Skin Ulcers

Warts

Neuro-emotional Usage:

Shock - especially when used with cinnamon.

Emotional Effect: Overwhelming (see neuro-emotional usage). It would take something this overwhelming to put a vampire at bay (good for young dating girls).

Contraindications: Low blood pressure. Do not use Neat garlic oil directly on the skin or ingest garlic oil Neat.

General Information:

The properties of garlic as the great 'anti' are ledgion. Suffice it to say that if it has anything to do with germs, bugs or parasites that are not friendly to living tissue, then garlic is going to do a house-cleaning job. Even though garlic doesn't really have an appreciated aromatherapy value as far as the Neuro-emotional is concerned, I've included it because of the other uses to aromatherapy (and herbology) it has.

Geranium (*Pelargonium graveolens*)

Classification: Cooling.

Best Source: Madagascar or Egypt.

Plant Part(s): Leaves.

Aroma: Light, rose like, and blossomy.

General Usage:

Adaptogenic Stimulant (Estrogenic and Adrenal Stimulant)

Herpes (Topical)

Lymphatic Decongestant

(Especially Mammary Glands)

Skin Disorders (Dry/Eczema)

Vaginal/Uterine Tonic (As A Douche)

Specific Topical Usage:

Cuts

Eczema

General Cosmetic Skin Care

Oily Skin

Skin Inflammations

Tonic for Slow Healing Sores

Neuro-emotional Usage:

"Out-Of-Balance"

Depression

Feeling Invaded and/or Pressed Upon

Uptight

Emotional Effect: Harmonious, integrated and at-oneness.

Contraindications: Skin that copiously secretes oils
(chamomile is best for this condition). Estrogenic
(over production of estrogen) conditions. Anxiety
conditions or overly Type A individuals.

General Information:

Geranium is used in many premium (high-grade)
skin care products for women. It has a strongly
estrogenic effect. A breast oil consisting of bergamot
(3 parts), ylang ylang (1 part) and geranium (3 parts)
cut with almond or olive oil (in which the EO's blend
is 5 to 10 percent of the finished oil) that's thoroughly
massaged into the breast is said to noticeably increase
breast size. A topical preparation for herpes
(especially type 3) consists of a blend of Chamomile (1
part), sandalwood (1 part), tea tree (3 parts), lavender
(3 parts), grapefruit (3 parts), and geranium (6 parts).
Apply Neat to the affected area – Use sparingly
(meaning do not "glopp" on).

Ginger (*Zingiber officinale*)

Classification: Warming.

Best Source: S. India.

Plant Part(s): Root.

Aroma: Medium, woodish, warm, and lightly pungent.

General Usage:

Antiseptic (Mild)   Digestant (Stimulant)
Carminative   Febrifuge
Diarrhea   Flatulence

Specific Topical Usage:

Stimulates surface blood flow and metabolism.

Neuro-emotional Usage:

Argumentative   Heated and Angry
Feeling Like "A   Mentally Confused
   Pressure Cooker   Ready To Explode
   Ready to Blow Up"   Sensation Like "A Hot
Feeling Unheard – Not   Sensitive Flash
   Listened To   Point"

Emotional Effect: Grounding and cooling.

Contraindications: Constipation (spastic).

General Information:

Like cayenne, ginger is a systemic stimulant. But unlike cayenne, ginger is a cooler more sustained stimulant of the body, working through the digestive system itself. Ginger has an affinity for the urinary system, and hence the eliminative functions of the skin. People who have difficulty sweating can often correct this by the use of ginger. Whole ginger herb taken internally (tea, capsule, or shaved root) followed immediately by a hot bath to which is added 1 to 2 cups of apple cider vinegar and 6 to 8 drops of ginger. Sit back, relax and sweat. To make the bath more relaxing to the nervous system add 2 to 4 drops of lavender oil.

Grapefruit, Pink (*Citrus paradisi*)

Classification: Cooling.

Best Source: S. U.S. or Israel.

Plant Part(s): Fruit rind.

Aroma: Light, fruity, biting bitterness, and freshening.

General Usage:

Cellulitis   Obesity

Detoxifying

Edema (Water
    Retention)

Specific Topical Usage:

Herpes   Stimulates Surface
                                                    Metabolism.

Neuro-emotional Usage:

"Down-N-Out"   Feeling Old
    Feelings   Moody (Bi-Polar)

Emotional Effect: Positive outlook on life and youthful.

Contraindications: Dehydration. The internal use blend as mentioned below should only be taken for ten consecutive days and then four days off and so on for two months, then take a one-month holiday before resuming the regime.

General Information:

Grapefruit is an excellent adjunct to weight control when used with fennel. A Neat oil preparation for internal use of 1 part grapefruit and 2 parts fennel is prepared then taken 2 to 3 drops 10 minutes before a meal or prior to a snack. Reverse the parts (2 parts grapefruit and 1 part fennel) and take once between each meal with a glass of water. Grapefruit EO can be cut with almond oil and vigorously rubbed into areas where cellulite is present. For best results this must be done twice daily over a period of four to twelve weeks for results to be obvious. For herpes see geranium.

Juniper (*Juniperus communis*)

Classification: Warming.

Best Source: Yugoslavia.

Plant Part(s): Fruit.

Aroma: Medium, resinous, herby, lightly fruity, and penetrating.

General Usage:

Antiseptic

Atonic Skin Lesions

Diabetes

Difficult Menstrual Periods

Flatulence (Due To Improper Protein Digestion)

Urinary Tract

Specific Topical Usage:

Acne

Dermatitis

Eczema

Infections

Skin Cleanser

Varicose Veins

Neuro-emotional Usage:

Creepy and Crawly Sensations

Depression (Intermittent)

Feeling Paralyzed To Do Anything

Feeling Violated

"Frozen-In-My-Tracks,"

Malaise

"Stabbed-In-The-Back," Overly Vulnerable.

Worry

Emotional Effect: Centers and refreshes.

Contraindications: Juniper should not be used where kidney inflammation and infection is present (juniper is popularly indicated for infections, however most infections are accompanied by inflammation, for which juniper is definitely contra-indicated). Refer to Sandalwood, since it is cooling to the urinary system.

General Information:

Juniper is used for urinary insufficiency where there is not kidney inflammation or infection. It is extremely stimulating to the urinary tract due to its increasing surface blood circulation effects on those tissues. When used in conjunction with thyme it is one of the most powerful urinary stimulants known (see thyme). Juniper can also be used as a vaginal douche in a blend consisting of geranium (2 parts), ylang ylang (2 parts), bergamot (4 parts), thyme (1 part) and juniper (8 parts) that is mixed in a 101 degree solution of 25 percent apple cider vinegar and 75 percent purified water. Juniper is also a digestive aid to sluggish digestion. Two excellent digestive aids can be made by blending juniper (3 parts) with peppermint (2 parts), thyme (1 part) and lemon (2 parts), or blending juniper (2 parts) with ginger (1 part), cinnamon (1 part) and cardamom (2 parts). Take 2 to 4 drops during or immediately following a meal.

Lavender (*Lavendula officinalis*)

Classification: Cooling.

Best Source: France.

Plant Part(s): Flowers.

Aroma: Medium, herby, and freshening.

General Usage:

Analgesic

Anti-inflammatory

Antiseptic

Antispasmodic

Anti-Venom/Poison (Bites)

Cicatrizing (Stimulates Skin and Wound Healing without Scarring – The Best)

Headaches (Vaso-Constrictive)

Hypertension

Stings and Contact Dermatitis)

Vermifuge

Specific Topical Usage:

Alopecia (Hair Loss)

Burns

Dermatitis

Dry Skin

General Cosmetic Skin Care

Skin Tonic.

Neuro-emotional Usage:

Anxiety

Enervated

Extreme Frustration

Insomnia (Can't Stop Thinking Or Worrying)

Melancholia (Caused
By Burn-Out)
Mental Exhaustion

"Out Of Balance"
"Ready To Explode"
Uptight

Emotional Effect: Expansive, unbound and limitless.

Contraindications: Light sun-sensitive skin. Chronic depression. Vaso-dilated headaches.

Special Note: Lavender will bleach the skin if skin is exposed to the UV rays or direct sunlight after applying lavender or any blend containing lavender.

General Information:

One of the most luxurious things that can be done is to draw a full bath of warm water, add 1 to 2 cups of Epsom salt and 4 to 6 drops of lavender EO. Then just slip carefully into the water, closing the eyes and inhaling the relaxing aroma, and as you immerse yourself into the water all the stress and hassles of the day dissipate right out of you. For the more adventurous, try any one of the other oils described in the book with the lavender bath to give it your own personality, unique character and specific activating or relaxing response.

Lavender is one of the finest anti-inflammatory agents known, especially where sensitive tissues are concerned. It is an excellent bath aid for babies with galled bottoms (diaper rash). Put 2 to 3 drops in the water, let baby soak for at least 15 minutes and when baby is removed from water, pat but don't rub dry. Lavender baths will also calm a baby with colic, fevers, enervation or crankiness. It is one of the most powerful cicatrizing agents known (see chamomile). It is also one of the best burn antiseptic analgesics there is, often resulting in little or no scarring (see tea tree). Used with cinnamon oil it is one of the best sting and bite antidotes known (see cinnamon). As an emotional therapeutic agent it is especially valuable where high anxiety driven by insomnia is present.

Lemon (*Citrus limonum*)

Classification: Cooling.

Best Source: Italy or Brazil.

Plant Part(s): Fruit rind.

Aroma: Light, lemonish, freshening, and bright.

General Usage:

Alterative Tonic

Antiseptic

Astringent

Oily Skin

Specific Topical Usage:

Oily and Congested Skin

Skin Cleanser

Stimulates Excretion of Waste through Skin Pores

Varicose Veins

Neuro-emotional Usage:

"Down-N-Out" Feeling

"It Just Keeps Slipping Right Through My Hands"

Confused

Feeling "Old and Worn Out"

Lacking Hope

Lethargic

Emotional Effect: Mental clarity and renewed hope.

Contraindications: Pathogenic liver problems (due to the high terpine content – use sage instead) especially where liver's synthesizing capabilities are not working.

General Information:

Like the whole fruit, lemon EO is referred to as a balancing agent. It is one of the best gastrointestinal antiseptic agents there is. In cases of stomach flu or food poisoning, I mix thyme (1 drop) and lemon (3 drops) and mix with a cup of hot apple cider vinegar water (1/3 vinegar to 2/3 water) or a cup of hot lemon water (a half fresh lemon squeezed into hot water) and sip slowly over 15 to 20 minutes. Lemon is one of the most effective EO's for cutting the smell and moderating the effects of garlic. An excellent cardiovascular and systemic tonic blend consists of garlic (1 part) and lemon (6 parts), from which 1 to 2 drops is added to a teaspoon of olive oil and then consumed. It should be remembered that of all the citrus plants lemon contains the highest percentage of terpines. Therefore, prolonged topical or internal use is discouraged. Prolonged topical use can result in dermatitis. Terpines have a cumulative, building-up effect in the liver because they are metabolized slowly by that organ. Internal usage should be slight to moderate, never heavy.

Lemongrass (*Cymbopogon citratus*)

Classification: Cooling.

Best Source: Madagascar or China.

Plant Part(s): The grass-like leaves.

Aroma: Medium, lemon like, and hay like.

General Usage:

Antiseptic

Gastric Stimulant

Glactagogue
(Insufficient Breast
Milk)

Parasympathetic
Nervous Tonic

Topical Parasiticide

Specific Topical Usage:

Closes Large Pores

Oily Skin

Neuro-emotional Usage:

Feel Like A Morose
Dream Out Of
Control

Feeling "All Washed
Out"

"I-Feel-Like-Crying"
(Not Necessarily
Depression)

No "Get-Up-N-Go"

Sluggish

Trouble Concentrating

Emotional Effect: Refreshes mind and body.

Contraindications: Over stimulated
parasympathetic system. Postpartum blues.

General Information:

Lemongrass is a regulator of the parasympathetic nervous system. Lemongrass is very powerful glactagogue and should be used in combination with fennel (see fennel) to enrich and increase breast milk. As a parasympathetic tonic (increases tone of parasympathetic system and decreases the tone of the sympathetic) it is best used with marjoram (see marjoram). In any use lemongrass should not be used alone but as part of a blend, and then only in small amounts.

Marjoram (*Origanum majorana*)

Classification: Cooling.

Best Source: S. Spain or Hungary.

Plant Part(s): Herb.

Aroma: Heavyish, herbish, and warming.

General Usage:

Anaphrodisiac (Decreases Sexual Desire)

Antispasmodic

Calming (To the Point of Sedating)

Expectorant (Moisturizing)

Gastro-Intestinal Tonic

Headaches (Vaso-Constricting)

Parasympathetic Tonic

Specific Topical Usage:

Burns

Cuts

Scrapes

Sores

Wounds

Neuro-emotional Usage:

"Can't-Take-The-Weekend-Off"

Enervation (Over Stimulated Sympathetic Nervous System)

Feeling All "Boxed In"

Grief

High Anxiety Responses

Inability to Slow Down and Relax

Insomnia (Caused By Over Active Sympathetic and Under Active Parasympathetic Nervous System)

"I'm-All-Tied-Up-Right-Now"

Mental Instability (Bi-Polar Tendencies)

Followed by Mental Exhaustion

Nervous Debility

Tics (Repetitive Neuro-Muscular Disorders)

"Too-Much-Work-To-Do"

Emotional Effect: Balancing and centering.

Contraindications: Do not use during pregnancy. Over stimulated parasympathetic system. Chronic depression. Vaso-dilated headaches.

General Information:

Marjoram is one of the most important herbs in cooking strong red meats that have been 'gamed.' In combination with other compatible EO's it can be one of the most powerful parasympathetic stimulants known. In cases of extreme hysteria bordering on shock (that's caused by over stimulation of the sympathetic nervous system) the following emergency EO's blend is very effective, even as an inhalant. Mix a blend of rose (1 part), lavender (3 parts), lemongrass (3 parts), and marjoram (4 parts). In an emergency apply Neat to the temples, behind the ears and massage into the neck muscles along the spineous-process, periodically cupping the hand (which now has the blend on it) and placing it over the affected persons nose to breath in the aroma. After a hard driving stress ridden day marjoram (3 drops) used with lavender (2 drops) and rose (1 drop) in an Epsom salt bath prior to retiring for the night is an excellent way to relax the body and mind prior to sleep.

Nutmeg (*Myristica fragrans*)

Classification: Cooling.

Best Source: West Indies.

Plant Part(s): Fruit (nut seed)

Aroma: Light, spicy, and biting.

General Usage:

Antiseptic

Lethargy

Malaise (Physical)

Oral/Toothaches

Rheumatic Muscle Conditions

Slow Metabolism

Specific Topical Usage: None.

Neuro-emotional Usage:

Atonic conditions of the body and mind

Fatigue

Mental and emotional confusion

Emotional Effect: Clarifies and enlivens.

Contraindications: Do not use during pregnancy. Nutmeg is a narcotic of which the fatal dosage (death) is concurrent with the hallucinogenic dose. Use externally only.

General Information:

I have included nutmeg for external use only, both as to its physiological applications and neuro-

emotional uses. It makes for a fine "nutmeg butter" that is used for toothaches and oral pains. A 'pseudo' nutmeg butter can be made by taking 1 ounce of pure creamed raw almond butter (no added salt, no roasting, etc.) and adding clove (2 drops) and nutmeg (4 to 6 drops). Kids will like this one; just remember that it needs to be kept in the mouth on the local sore spot as long a possible. This same butter blend can be turned into a rheumatic rub by adding rosemary (4 drops) to the butter and massaging into the affected muscles or joints.

Patchouli (*Pogostemon patchouli*)

Classification: Cooling.

Best Source: Madagascar or Indonesia.

Plant Part(s): Leaves.

Aroma: Heavy, woody, musty, sensuous, and very earthy.

General Usage:

Anti-Fungal (One of the Best)

Anti-inflammatory

Antiseptic

Chapped Skin

Mildly Cicatrizing (Skin and Wound Healer)

Moth Repellent (Put on Cedar Chips)

Specific Topical Usage:

Aging Skin

Closes Purulent Wounds

General Skin Care

Wrinkles

Neuro-emotional Usage:

"All Washed Out"

Depression (Chronic)

Floating

Lack Of Self Esteem

Low Libido

Mental Fatigue

Ungrounded

Emotional Effect: Confidence and charisma.

Contraindications: People who have a highly melancholic personality.

General Information:

Patchouli is most known as being the consummate "hippie" perfume and was used extensively in incense sticks, sensuous massage oils and unguents. To the international traveler of yesteryear patchouli was applied to hankies and liberally placed throughout one's luggage as it was an excellent moth repellent (not to mention that it served notice to whoever they were staying with that they were a person who was well traveled).

Patchouli{ XE "Patchouli" } is now receiving more recognition as one of the best anti-fungal agents known. An excellent preparation for foot fungus is a blend of chamomile (1 part) and patchouli (4 parts) cut with hemp oil (EO blend is 10 percent of the finished oil) then applied directly to the affected part and covered with a white cotton sock. Wear only sandals so the fresh air can also do its part until the condition corrects itself. If the situation is extremely serious and this blend is only partially effective, the inclusion of cinnamon (1 part) to the above blend can be done, but be warned, it will be a very prickly hot experience. Even so, this will usually take care of the most serous cases of foot fungus.

Peppermint (*Mentha piperita*)

Classification: Warming.

Best Source: Willamette valley of Oregon or N. Idaho, U.S.

Plant Part(s): Herb.

Aroma: Medium, mintish, bitterish, penetrating, and sweetish.

General Usage:

Analgesic

Antiseptic

Antispasmodic

Congestion

Digestant

Headaches (Vaso-Constrictive)

Remineralizer

Specific Topical Usage:

Acne

Congested Skin Conditions

Invigorates Tired Skin

Refreshing Hair Rinse

Neuro-emotional Usage:

Episodes of Fainting

Feelings of A Lost Youth

Hysteria

Lack of Mental Concentration

Malaise

Wasting Away

Emotional Effect: Invigorating and cooling.

Contraindications: Do not take at same time as homeopathic remedies.

General Information:

Everyone is familiar with peppermint, the aroma and smell of red and white Christmas candy canes. Or a sprig (leaf or short leaf stem) placed in a glass of summer ice tea (preferably herbal of course) or lemonade. Peppermint is the mint of "Ahh..." It refreshes and enlivens the senses. Commonly, it conjures up the idyllic easy days of summer when we were young and free. Peppermint applied and rubbed into the temples has relieved many a headache, particularly vaso-constrictive ones. Peppermint has a special affinity for potassium and is known as one of the best mineral electrolyte remineralizers there is. It stimulates gastric activity while balancing acid/alkaline balance –especially when used with Lemon). A fabulous digestive aid & remineralizer can be made by mixing a blend of lemon (1 part) and peppermint (1 part). Use 2 to 4 drops taken sometime during or immediately following a meal. Blending tea tree (2 parts) and peppermint (1 part) can make a refreshing hair rinse.

Pine (*Pinus sylvestris*)

Classification: Cooling.

Best Source: Russia (Siberia).

Plant Part(s): Wood.

Aroma: Medium, clarified, and balsamic.

General Usage:

Antiseptic

Balances Circulation

Decongestant

Expectorant

Specific Topical Usage:

Foot odors

Neuro-emotional Usage:

"Down-N-Out" Feeling

Anxiety

Emotionally Weak

Feeling Polluted

Flighty

Lack Of Concentration

Mental Fatigue

Emotional Effect: Refreshing and invigorating.

Contraindications: Overly dry respiratory conditions.

General Information:

Pine is a cooling scent that has the refreshing qualities of being in the middle of a pine forest following a summer shower. Similar to eucalyptus in its air purifying qualities, pine has a gentle ionizing effect. It is excellent for dealing with anxiety situations. For general air purification purposes using an aromatherapy diffuser it is excellent when cut with eucalyptus and a small amount of tea tree oil.

Rose Moroc Clear (*Rosa damascena varietal*)

Classification: Cooling.

Best Source: Morocco.

Plant Part(s): Flowers (petals).

Aroma: Heavy, blossomy, and wandering.

General Usage:

Antiseptic

Antispasmodic

Chaffed Skin

Cooling to the Skin as a 'Rose Water'

Drying Skin (Stimulates Sebaceous Oil Production)

Nervous Tonic

Soothing Astringent

Spleen Tonic

Specific Topical Usage:

Bruises

Eczema

General Skin Care

Inflamed Skin (From Skin Allergies)

Skin Care for Babies

Tonic and Cooling to Skin

Neuro-emotional Usage:

Anger (Driven by Suppressed Grief or Betrayal)

Depression (Chronic)

Grief

Loss
Low Libido

Unrequited Love and
Affection

Emotional Effect: Endearment and hope.

Contraindications: High anxiety profiles.

General Information:

Special Note: I have listed Rose Moroc Clear instead of Rose Bulgarian because of its availability and safe and effective ease of use. To make 1 ounce of Rose Bulgarian, also known as rose otto (distilled) or rose absolute (solvent extracted) requires hundreds of pounds of Bulgarian rose petals and a lengthy manufacturing process, hence the high cost, which is over $2,000.00 per ounce on the open market.

Rose is one of the most heady scents known, matched only by jasmine. And no wonder, they are two of the most expensive EO's available and both require extremely small amounts to gain the anticipated effect, whether for physiological or emotional responses. It is one of the best aromas for chronic depression available. A blend consisting of ylang ylang (1 part), bergamot (4 parts) and rose (1 part) serves as an excellent all around anti-depressant aroma. Rose can be mixed with a commercially available witch hazel lotion (3 to 4 drops per 8 ounces of witch hazel) that will make it a very soothing 'modified rose water' lotion for dry chaffed skin and prickly heat.

Rosemary (*Rosmarinus officinalis*)

Classification: Warming.

Best Source: S. Spain.

Plant Part(s): Herb.

Aroma: Medium, camphor like, woody, and biting.

General Usage:

Antiseptic

Digestant (Stimulates Fatty Acid Digestion)

Male Pattern Balding

Oily Skin and Hair

Respiratory Problems

Stiff And Sore Muscles

Specific Topical Usage:

Hair Loss

Oily Skin

Skin Parasites

Used In Dark Hair Rinses

Neuro-emotional Usage:

Apathy

Bi-Polar (Mild)

Low View of Life

Melancholy

Memory Loss

Spiritually Depressed

Emotional Effect: Refreshing and clarification.

Contraindications: Overactive digestion. Dry chaffed skin.

General Information:

Rosemary is best known as the 'hair herb.' It is particularly indicated for people with limp greasy hair and an oily scalp that often contributes to balding problems. An excellent hair rinse can be made consisting of one pint of warm apple cider vinegar to which 4 to 6 drops of rosemary is added. After shampooing, first rinse out the shampoo with the regular water. When the shampoo is removed then apply the warm rosemary vinegar hair rinse and let stand for a minute then rinse the rosemary vinegar hair rinse out.

Rosemary is also one of the best fatty acid digestive aids there is. A specific digestive aid can be made by blending lemon (1 part), thyme (1 part) and rosemary (3 parts) and taking 2 to 4 drops with or immediately following a fatty rich meal. A deep heating and penetrating muscle rub is made by blending eucalyptus (4 parts), cajeput (2 parts), thyme (1 part) and rosemary (4 parts) which is cut with a fixed oil (EO blend being 25 percent of the final oil) and vigorously massage it into the affected muscle group.

Sandalwood (*Santalum album*)

Classification: Cooling.

Best Source: Mysore region of India.

Plant Part(s): Wood.

Aroma: Heavy, woodish, sweet, and balsamic.

General Usage:

Antiseptic

Antispasmodic

Bronchitis

Dry Skin

Expectorant (Drying)

Lack of Libido

Urinary Tract

Specific Topical Usage:

Acne

Dry Skin

Eczema

General Skin Care

Rejuvenates Skin

Neuro-emotional Usage:

Anxiety

Closed to Emotions

Ego-Centricity

Lack of Sexual Awareness

Low Self Image

Overly Grounded (Cynical)

Repressed (But not Depressed) Emotions

Spiritually Empty

Emotional Effect: Relaxing and centering.

Contraindications: Overly spiritualized (cloud bouncers). Overly open and revealing of own personal feelings ("tell all"-ers).

General Information:

Sandalwood is an excellent urinary tract antiseptic that does not irritate like juniper does. In cases of infectious inflammation it is one of the best, however, a little goes a long, long way. Sandalwood is one of the most potent of all aromas, which also is an indication of its strength. Recommended is 1 to 2 drops of sandalwood in a teaspoon of honey slowly swallowed and chased with a cup of warm (not hot) marsh mallow tea. Every other time add 1 drop of thyme to the sandalwood/honey mixture. This is done two times a day for 3 to 4 days only.

As for the emotional therapy use of sandalwood, there is a tradition coming out of the East that if one wears sandalwood essence they will attract the spiritually inclined and put off the unspiritually inclined. I've tried this a number of times and must say that there is some basis for this belief.

Tea Tree (*Maleleuca alternifolia*)

Classification: Warming.

Best Source: Australia.

Plant Part(s): Leaves.

Aroma: Medium, medicinal, sharp, penetrating, and freshening.

General Usage:

Anti-Fungal
Anti-inflammatory
Antiseptic
Antiviral
Bites and Stings

Respiratory (Expanding Warmth)
Serious Burns

Specific Topical Usage:

Acne
Fungal Infections

Stimulates Scalp Circulation

Neuro-emotional Usage:

Hysteria
Panic

Unclean Feelings

Emotional Effect: Cleansing and light.

Contraindications: Dried mucous membranes.

General Information:

Tea Tree is one of the most popular single EO's on the market today. It is one of the few EO's here in the United States that has been as well researched and clinically investigated as the dozens of EO's have been in Europe. Because of this it is one of the most commercially developed EO's for consumer products in the U.S. Soaps, shampoos, conditioners, lotions, massage oils, etc. have all been developed and marketed to the public at large. It is from the same family as eucalyptus. However, tea tree oil has many therapeutic advantages eucalyptus does not provide. The most prominent is that less people show a sensitivity to tea tree than eucalyptus, and it is 'cleaner' feeling as well. Because it contains a lower amount of resinoid producing components, tea tree is more suited to consumer product development than eucalyptus.

In cases of a sore scratchy throat 2 drops of tea tree in a teaspoonful of honey swallowed slowly is a good remedy. Do this every two to three hours for a day. An anti-inflammatory/antiseptic burn preparation can be made by blending lavender (1 part) with tea tree (2 parts) and then adding 6 to 8 drops of the EO blend with 8 ounces of Rose water in a sterilized spray bottle. Spray a light layer of the water on the burns every 30 minutes to an hour. It keeps the wound cool, germ free, properly moisturized, relatively pain free and promotes tissue healing. Another EO blend for bites and stings can be made by blending cinnamon/lavender (see cinnamon). Blend (2 parts) with tea tree (1 part).

Thyme, Red (*Thymus vulgaris*)

Classification: Warming.

Best Source: S. Spain or Egypt.

Plant Part(s): Herb.

Aroma: Heavy, biting, penetrating, sweet, and medicinal.

General Usage:

Anti-Fungal

Antiseptic

Antispasmodic

Antiviral

Digestant (Stimulates Fatty and Protein Digestion)

Expectorant (Drying)

Menstruation Aid

Upper Respiratory Aid

Urinary Problems

Specific Topical Usage:

Antiseptic for Wounds

Athletes Foot

Fungal Infections

Mouth & Gum Care

Neuro-emotional Usage:

"Gotta-Stay-on-Schedule-or..."

Anxiety

Feeling Pressured

Frustration

Lethargic

Mentally Fatigued

Mildly Enervated

Emotional Effect: Clarity (mental) and enlivened.

Contraindications: Dried pulmonary system.

General Information:

Thyme is an excellent warming digestive aid (see juniper). It has very powerful antiviral agents that are some of the strongest seen in any EO. An airborne disinfecting aromatherapy diffuser blend can be made (see eucalyptus) that will kill airborne bacteria, viruses, germs and have an expectorant action on the lungs. Thyme has both a gentle stimulating and aggressive stimulating action on the urinary system. This is determined by what it is blended with. If blended with sandalwood it will have a gentle stimulating action that is non-irritating (see sandalwood). If blended with juniper, say thyme (1 part) and juniper (2 parts); it will result in one of the most powerful urinary stimulants there is. It is a very good EO in a vaginal douche acting as a catalyst to the other EO's in the blend (see juniper). It's also a very good digestive antiseptic for stomach flu and food poisoning (see lemon).

Ylang Ylang Extra (*Canaga odorata*)

Classification: Cooling.

Best Source: Madagascar.

Plant Part(s): Flowers.

Aroma: Strongly heavy, heady, blossomy, and sweet.

General Usage:

Antispasmodic
Cardio-Tonic
Hypertension

Lack Of Libido (For Women Specifically)

Specific Topical Usage:

Aging Skin
Oily

Stimulates Breast Growth

Neuro-emotional Usage:

"Life-Is-A-Walk-Down-A-Dark-Damp-Foggy-Lane"
Depression (Chronic)
Down on Self

Hopelessness
Icy Coldness towards Others
Inability to Love Self
Rage

Emotional Effect: Openness and caring.

Contraindications: Do not use on people with anxiety Type A profiles or tendencies towards manic behavior.

General Information:

Ylang ylang is another heady aroma. A little goes a long, long way. It is an excellent cardio-tonic, especially when used with hawthorn tea. One drop of ylang ylang EO to a full cup of hawthorn tea two to four (no more) times a week is an excellent enhancement to this well proven and time honored cardio-tonic herb.

Sample Aromatherapy Blends

The following are sample, "do-it-yourself" blends you can use for various purposes. All blends are given in parts. A part can be whatever quantity you desire, such as one drop or one ounce depending on the amount of the blend you wish to make.

Antiseptic/Disinfecting Blends

The following blends are for killing microorganisms and fighting infection. A few may be used internally. Most are for topical use.

Four Thieves Vinegar

As promised, here is the actual recipe for the "Vinegar of the Four Thieves" also known as "Marseilles vinegar." This aromatic antiseptic vinegar is a specific for contagious diseases. It's rubbed on the body, put in small bottles to be sniffed and in the absence of a nebulizing diffuser can be heated to boiling temperature to diffuse into and throughout the room.

> 3 pints of strong white wine vinegar (do not use brown vinegar as it will offset the aromatic character of the essential oils components of the herbs).

1 handful each of wormwood, meadowsweet,
    juniper berries, wild marjoram and sage
50 cloves
2 ounces of elecampane root
2 ounces of angelica
2 ounces of rosemary
2 ounces of horehound
3 grams camphor

Blend the ingredients into the vinegar and steep for 10 days. After the 10 days strain the herbs and filter the fluid through several layers of cheesecloth or other fine cloth.

Emergency Disinfectant

This blend is for carrying in an emergency kit. In an emergency it is added to water for disinfecting a wound or used Neat to clean a knife where no fire or alcohol is available, and it can be applied Neat to a bandage and the bandage applied directly to a wound.

Tea tree	4 parts
Lavender	2 parts
Rose	2 parts

Pocket Hand Antiseptic

This blend is carried in a purse or pocket. Prior to dealing with a pathological situation massage this blend into the hands prior to washing hands, then wash hands with soap. After completing task, wash hands, and then repeat first cycle. This regime also has the added benefit of moisturizing the hands.

Lavender	6 parts
Eucalyptus	4 parts
Thyme	1 part
Fixed Oil	180 parts

Mix EO's with blend with fixed oil at 5 to 7 percent of finished product.

Strong Disinfectant

This blend is for adding to a cleaning solution. Add 10 to 20 drops of the Neat blend per gallon of cleaning solution to use as a disinfectant.

Bergamot	4 parts
Clove	2 parts
Pine	2 parts
Cinnamon	1 parts
Thyme	1 part

Citrus Deodorizer

A blend for eliminating cooking or offensive odors that can be inhaled from the bottle, put in an aromatherapy diffuser or 8 to 10 drops in a pan of water and brought to a boil to infuse throughout the room.

| Grapefruit | 4 parts |

Lemon	4 parts
Rosemary	1 part

"Fresh Air" Deodorizer

A blend for eliminating cooking or offensive odors that can be inhaled from the bottle, put in an aromatherapy diffuser or 8 to 10 drops in a pan of water and brought to a boil to infuse throughout the room.

Lemon	6 parts
Rosemary	3 parts
Nutmeg	1 part

Blends for Specific Health Problems

The following blends are designed to aid specific health problems.

Hypertension Blend

Used to help regulate hypertension. Inhaled throughout the day from the bottle. Add two drops to a glass of herbal tea indicated for hypertension.

Marjoram	2 parts
Lavender	1 part
Ylang ylang	1 part

Aromatic Weight Control

Has the effect of eliminating excess fluid from the body and mildly deterring the appetite. Inhale from the bottle when a snack-attack hits or when hungry. Put 2 to 4 drops in a glass of warm fresh squeezed lemon water three times a day also helps.

Grapefruit	4 parts
Lemon	1 part
Juniper	1 part

Cellulite Dissolver

3 drops four times a day in a stout oriental green tea (or green matte) three times a week, used for several months.

Grapefruit	4 drops
Lemon	2 drops
Juniper	2 drops

Fever Reducer

Breathe a number of times, put on pulse points, across eye-brows, then go to bed to recuperate.

Peppermint	3 parts
Eucalyptus	2 parts
Bergamot	1 part
Pine	1 part

Minty Digestive Settler

For nausea, vomiting and mild digestive problems. Inhale from the bottle. If that doesn't work, add 2 to 3 drops to ice cold water and sip very, very slowly in small sips until the problem passes.

Peppermint	3 parts
Fennel	1 part

Hangover Helper

For the morning after. It settles and balances the stomach's buffering system, which results in a refreshing reflex action throughout the rest of the body and lifts the heavy hangover feeling.

Fennel	1 part
Peppermint	1 part

"Sweeten the Breath" Mouthwash

For bad breath (halitosis) as a mouthwash. Mix 6 drops with a small cup of salt water and gargle vigorously.

Bergamot	1 parts
Lemon	1 parts
Peppermint	1 part

Oral Antiseptic

For gum care (as a mouthwash w/salt & baking soda). Mix 4 drops with mouthwash, gargle and hold in mouth for a few long moments before expelling.

Peppermint	2 parts
Thyme	1 part

Chamomile & Rosemary Hair Care

As a hair rinse – 4 to 8 drops per pint of warm water. The same 4 to 8 drops works even better in a pint of warm brown vinegar.

Chamomile	2 parts
Rosemary	2 parts
Rose	1 part
Sage	1 part

Overactive Digestive Aid

Take 2 to 4 drops on the tongue and swallow slowly. This blend should only be used for overactive digestion (acidic).

Lemon	2 parts
Bergamot	1 part
Peppermint	1 part

Underactive Digestive Aid

Mix 3 to 5 drops with a teaspoon of honey and ingest prior to a meal. This blend (and the honey) should not be used with overactive digestion.

Chamomile	2 parts
Ginger	2 parts
Sage	1 part
Peppermint	1 part

Digestive Antispasmodic

For gastric spasms. Take 1 oz of fixed oil, add 10 to 12 drops and gently rub on the abdomen and take 2 drops on the tongue and slowly swallow.

Chamomile	4 parts
Lavender	2 parts
Rose	2 parts
Rosemary	1 part

Carminative

For flatulence. Take 3 to 4 drops with a warm glass of lightly salted water (sea salt or real salt) and slowly drink and relax until wind is expelled.

Peppermint	3 parts
Sage	1 part
Ginger	1 part
Thyme	1 part

Aromatic Blends for Children

The following blends are designed to help with health problems experienced by babies and children.

Colic and Sleep Aid Bath

Relieves colic and induces sleep (put 2 to 4 drops in warm bath water).

Lavender	2 parts
Chamomile	1 part

Rashes and Chaffing Bath

Antiseptic/healing – rashes and chaffing (put 2 to 4 drops in warm bath water).

Lemon	3 parts
Lavender	2 parts
Chamomile	1 part

"Nighttime" Cold and Flu Aid

Colds or flu (put 4 to 6 drops on pillow or hanky inserted between pillow and pillow case).

Eucalyptus	1 part
Tea tree	1 part
Lavender	1 part

Earache Oil

Earaches – congested. Applied as 20 percent of a fixed oil base (2 to 3 drops in each ear).

Cajeput	1 part
Lavender	1 part
Fixed Oil	20 parts

Antiseptic Earache Oil

Same directions as above except only 1 to 2 drops in each ear. Stronger antiseptic action.

Lavender	6 parts
Cajeput	4 part
Garlic	1 part

Toothache Relief

Applied as 20 percent of a fixed oil base directly to the affected tooth and gum.

Cajeput	2 parts
Rose	2 parts
Clove	1 part
Fixed Oil	20 parts

"Clear the Congestion" Pillows

Respiratory infection and congestion (4 to 8 drops as an inhalant on bed pillow)

Eucalyptus	2 parts
Lavender	2 parts
Tea tree	1 part

Tummy Soothe

Soothing tummy massage oil (as 7 percent of fixed oil base).

Chamomile	5 parts
Ginger	2 parts
Peppermint	3 parts
Nutmeg	1 part
Fixed oil	140 parts

Blends for Teenagers/Young Adults

The following formulas are designed especially for problems experienced by teenagers and young adults.

Great-Looking Skin Care Wash

General skin care/toning (for bath or washbasin use 4 to 6 drops).

| Chamomile | 3 parts |

Geranium	1 part
Rose	1 part

"Before that Date" Deodorizing Bath

Deodorizing bath (used with bath water while taking a soap-cleaning bath – 4 drops applied directly to soapy lathered wash cloth).

Lemongrass	4 parts
Rosemary	4 parts
Chamomile	2 parts
Citronella	1 part

"Zap that Zit" Acne Wash

Acne/blemish facial wash (used in washbasin for washing face – 4 to 6 drops).

Rose	5 parts
Chamomile	2 parts
Tea tree	1 part

Aromatic Blends for Women

The following formulas are designed for problems experienced by women.

"That Time of the Month" Oil

PMS reliever with a diuretic action. Use 4 drops in bath water and/or as a vaginal douche use 4 to 6 drops per 24 oz douche.

Rosemary	7 parts
Juniper	5 parts
Geranium	2 parts
Sandalwood	1 part

Marjoram Menstrual Aid

Brings on period by putting 2 to 4 drops in bath.

Marjoram	2 parts
Sage	2 parts
Rose	1 part

Bergamot Blue's Buster

For post menstrual or partum blues put 3 to 5 drops in bath.

Bergamot	4 parts
Lemongrass	1 part
Rose	1 part

Sitz Bath Blend

Hip bath (especially after lengthy blood loss period). Use 4 to 8 drops in hip bath water.

Geranium	3 parts
Rose	2 parts
Sandalwood	1 part

Vaginal Douche

For clearing up discharges. Use 4 to 8 drops in 24 ounces of water or a cooling and astringing tea blend.

Sage	2 parts
Geranium	1 part
Rose	1 part

Get Rid of the "Yeastie Beasties" Douche

For control of vaginal yeast (candida) use the following blend in a douche. Put 8 drops into 24 oz of liquid. Yarrow, calendula and/or chaparral tea make a good liquid base. Use twice daily.

Bergamot	3 parts
Chamomile	2 parts
Geranium	2 parts
Lavender	2 parts
Tea tree	3 parts
Thyme	1 part

Blends for Emotional Problems

The following blends are for various emotional problems. Remember that some individuals may have different emotional responses than the majority of individuals.

Shock Blend

To be smelled and applied to pulse points.

Marjoram	3 parts
Rose	3 parts
Ylang ylang	2 parts
Sandalwood	1 part
Pine	1 part
Sage	1 part
Thyme	1 part

Shock Blend Two

A more direct shock blend that is not only applied to pulse points but is also inhaled from the bottle.

Rose	2 parts
Ylang ylang	2 parts
Sage	1 part

Mental Clarity

Helps clear the mind of fogginess and clarifies the incoming ambient light through the visual cortex. Inhale from the bottle.

Bergamot	4 parts
Lemon	2 parts
Lemongrass	1 part

Mental Clarity Two

Used in place of the previous blend. Inhale from the bottle.

Lavender	2 parts
Patchouli	1 part
Rose	1 part

Malaise Fighter

For feelings of general sickness or malaise (best described as a kind of overall "yucky" feeling). Use as an inhalant and on temples, ears and eyebrows.

Peppermint	3 parts
Ginger	2 part
Ylang ylang	1 part

Adrenal Support

Formula which tonifies and stimulates the adrenals. Best used by simply inhaling throughout the day from the bottle. Can be added to an adrenal strengthening tea (1 to 2 drops).

Lavender	1 part
Pine	3 parts

Pancreatic Support

For strengthening and tonifying the pancreas. Use as 7 percent of a fixed oil base and rub into the middle back (kidney area). Can be added to a pancreatic strengthening tea (1 to 2 drops).

Bergamot	1 part
Ginger	1 part
Juniper	2 parts

Aromatic Massage Oils

A good fixed massage oil base consists of almond, olive or cold pressed hemp oil (80 percent); cut with grape seed oil (10 Percent) and another light viscosity vegetable oil (10 percent) of your choosing (peanut, safflower, etc.). This is your 100 percent fixed oil base to which you will add any of the following EO blends. The EO blends will be 5 to 15 percent of the finished massage oil blend. Add the percentage (5 to 15 percent) of EO blend according your discretion.

"Ease the Pain" Massage Blend

General pain relieving blend.

Marjoram	5 parts
Lavender	4 parts
Ginger	4 parts
Chamomile	3 parts
Juniper	3 parts
Nutmeg	1 part
Fixed oil	Calculate

Rheumatism Rub

For massaging into painful joints as an aid for rheumatism.

Juniper	2 parts
Rosemary	2 parts
Lavender	1 part
Lemon	1 part
Ginger	1 part
Fixed oil	Calculate

Invigorating Massage Blend

For enlivening the senses of the body.

Bergamot	4 parts

Rosemary	2 parts
Ylang ylang	1 part
Juniper	1 part
Fixed oil	Calculate

Invigorating Massage Blend Two

A variant on the previous blend.

Bergamot	5 parts
Rosemary	2 parts
Fixed oil	Calculate

Relaxing Massage Blend

For relaxing the senses of the body.

Lavender	14 parts
Sandalwood	8 parts
Chamomile	4 part
Patchouli	2 parts
Nutmeg	1 part

"Laid-Back" Lavender Massage Blend

A variant on the previous blend.

Lavender	6 parts
Chamomile	2 parts
Rose	1 part

Relaxing Rose Massage Blend

Another variant on the previous two blends.

Rose	7 parts
Lavender	5 parts
Geranium	1 part

Bergamot Balancing Massage Oil

For balancing and centering the senses of the body.

Bergamot	6 part
Rosemary	2 parts
Lavender	2 parts
Sage	1 part

A Must for the Bust

Now, you may laugh at or find the following unbelievable, but it really works. It's a massage blend for 'bust growth.' Many women experience small busts because either the supporting muscles are uptight and restricting adequate blood flow to the breast or the lymphatics themselves are so slow moving that adequate nutritional exchange for bust growth is hindered. The massage alone helps immensely. But when used with the following bust growth enhancing EO blends not only is circulation enhanced, but there is a subtle hormonal response as well due to the EO's being absorbed into the body at this point of application. These specific EO's have been found to be hormonally responsive in women. I recommend mixing this blend at 10 percent of the finished massage oil blend. The massaging with these EO's should be done every day for the first month and then two to three times a week thereafter.

Geranium	2 parts
Ylang ylang	3 parts

Another Breast Enhancer

Here's another formula that aids breast development.

Geranium	2 parts
Ylang ylang	3 parts
Fennel	1 part

Massage Oils for Romantic Nights

The following massage oils are perfect for a romantic evening with your partner.

Loving Mood Massage Oil

To soften and romanticize the emotions.

Rose	4 parts
Sandalwood	1 part

Patchouli Passion Massage Oil

A his and her blend that specifically opens and balances male and female emotional energy flow.

Patchouli	2 parts
Sandalwood	1 part

Sensuous Moments Massage Oil

For sensualizing and soothing the senses and emotions.

Rose	3 parts
Geranium	1 part

Romantic Roses Massage Oil

Another blend for creating a sensuous, loving mood with your partner.

Rose	4 parts
Lavender	2 part
Ylang ylang	1 part (optional)

More Suggestions for Passion Boosters

Patchouli and sandalwood oils by themselves are great. Don't use more than 5 percent of these two oils by themselves however. As a general rule, the patchouli seems to assuage the masculine energies, whereas the sandalwood seems to assuage the feminine energies. They are best used together due to the fact that traditionally patchouli is a grounding scent whereas sandalwood is a lifting ethereal scent. Used together they act as a wholeness based single scent.

Aromatic Foot Baths

Aromatic foot baths are not only relaxing they're very therapeutic as well. The feet are very absorptive. The following foot bath blends are recommended for common foot problems. Fill a pan with water (tepid or warm depending on the blend) so that the water will reach the ankles. Add six to twelve drops of the blends to the water and soak the feet for 15 to 20 minutes.

"Fungus Amugus" Foot Soak

For athlete's foot and other foot or toe nail fungus problems.

Tea tree	6 parts
Garlic	2 part
Sandalwood	1 part

Foot Fungus Fighter

Here's another foot bath for athlete's foot.

Tea tree	6 parts
Patchouli	2 parts
Garlic	2 part
Thyme	2 parts

A Neat Treat for Sweaty Feet

This formula actually acts as an antiperspirant for the feet. It helps to reduce sweating in the feet and prevent odor.

Pine	2 part
Lavender	1 part
Sage	1 part

"Oh, My Aching Feet" Relief

A soothing foot bath for tired and aching feet.

Rosemary	2 parts
Juniper	1 part

More Relief for Tired Feet

Another foot bath which relaxes and soothes those tired, sore feet.

Chamomile	1 part
Lavender	1 part
Juniper	2 parts

Aromatic Bath Oil Blends

For aromatic baths use Neat oils (pure undiluted oils as described in Chapter Three). Put 4 to 8 drops of the blend in standing bath water. When dealing with tired aching muscles add Epsom salts to bath water. The oils can also be added directly to Epsom salts to make your own bath salts. Add about 4 to 8 drops of the oil blend to a cup of Epsom salts.

"Coffee Substitute" Stimulating Bath

A stimulating bath blend to help you get going in the morning.

Bergamot	2 parts
Pine	1 part
Rosemary	2 parts

Morning "Wake-up Call"

Feeling sluggish? This one act like a gentle massage to the nervous system.

Ylang ylang	1 part
Bergamot	2 parts

Pine Forest Morning

A refreshing bath for balmy mornings and heavy feelings.

Pine	2 parts
Rosemary	1 part

"Lemon Scrub" Cleansing Bath

A disinfectant and antiseptic bath which also helps to clear and refresh the mind.

Lemon	3 parts
Geranium	1 part
Pine	1 part

Pine & Lemon Cleansing Bath

A variant on the previous blend.

Pine	1 part
Lemon	1 part

Geranium & Sandalwood Cleansing Bath

Another variant on the previous two blends.

Geranium	1 part
Sandalwood	1 part

"Laid Back" Lavender Soak

A relaxing bath blend for muscular stress and tension. Add to the bath with Epsom salts for very best effect.

Lavender	2 parts
Marjoram	2 parts
Rose	1 part

Unwind After that Hard Day at the Office

A blend that counters the emotional effects of a harried day at the office (or at home for the mothers).

Chamomile	2 parts
Marjoram	2 parts
Rose	1 part

"Give me a Sedative, Please?" Bath

For insomnia. If you can't get to sleep, run a warm bath (not too hot) and soak for twenty minutes. Pat dry with the towel and go back to bed.

Chamomile	2 parts
Lavender	2 parts
Nutmeg	1 part

Special Blends for Diffusers

I recommend that eucalyptus be exclusively used as the sole cutting agent for EO's used in nebulizing diffusers. In each of the following diffuser blends I've listed eucalyptus as a percentage. This means that eucalyptus by itself represents that percentage of the finished EO blend being put into the nebulizer. Over the years I have found eucalyptus to be the best single EO cutting agent and carrier for this task. It also meets all the antiseptic and disinfecting criteria. You can experiment with the percentage of eucalyptus used, even discarding its addition to a blend altogether (except for the antiseptic/disinfecting blends). Not using it to cut a blend will require turning the diffuser pump up to full force and necessitate cleaning the nebulizer more often. Because it is a top note EO its aroma gives way to the other EO's in a blend.

Clean the Air

Nebulized air disinfectant. Pour Neat into nebulizer and then turn on diffuser.

Lavender	6 parts
Bergamot	3 parts
Juniper	2 parts
Tea tree	2 parts
Pine	1 part

Eucalyptus[8]   70 to 80 percent of blend

Sleep Easy

Nebulized blend for insomnia

Bergamot   2 parts
Lavender   2 parts
Rose   1 part
Eucalyptus   50 to 70 percent of blend

A Good Night's Rest

Turn on 30 minutes prior to going to bed and then turn off when you retire.

Chamomile   2 parts
Lavender   1 part
Eucalyptus   50 to 70 percent of blend

---

[8] to clean nebulizer after the heavier components of EO's have concentrated into bottom of a nebulizer, I recommend using eucalyptus itself as the sole cutting and cleaning agent. This helps maintain a adulterant free nebulizer. Of all the EO's it is usually the least expensive and it is the most effective EO to cut other EO's for diffuser use, since it decreases viscosity and increases the nubulizing effect while sustaining the individual EO's therapeutic characteristics as well.

Lavender Dreams

For those who sleep fitfully throughout the night. Turn on for 1 hour before bedtime and then turn off when you retire.

Lavender	2 parts
Rose	1 part (optional)
Eucalyptus	3-4 parts (50 to 70 percent)

"Infuse Me with Energy" Formula

Nebulized blends for lethargy or balminess — especially in the morning.

Juniper	2 parts
Pine	2 parts
Ylang ylang	1 part
Eucalyptus	6-8 parts (60 to 80 percent)

"Lift My Spirits" Diffuser Blend

Another energizing aromatherapy blend for diffusers.

Juniper	3 parts
Pine	2 parts
Ylang ylang	1 part
Patchouli	1 part
Eucalyptus	8-10 parts (60 to 80 percent)

Ylang Ylang Pick-Me-Up Blend

Another variation on the two previous blends.

Ylang ylang	2 part
Pine	1 part
Eucalyptus	4-9 parts (60 to 80 percent)

Romantic Evening

Nebulized blend for enhancing sensuous feelings.

Patchouli	2 parts
Rose	1 part
Eucalyptus	3-5 parts (50 to 70 percent)

"In the Mood for Love"

A nebulized blend for heady nights to be remembered.

Rose	3 parts
Sandalwood	1 part
Eucalyptus	50 to 70 percent of blend

"Light My Fire"

A blend that sensitizes the senses, especially for women.

| Rose | 6 parts |

Geranium	1 part
Ylang ylang	1 part
Eucalyptus	50 to 70 percent of blend

Passionate Desires

A relaxing blend that relieves tension and opens the senses.

Lavender	2 parts
Geranium	1 part
Ylang ylang	1 part
Eucalyptus	50 to 70 percent of blend

Bedroom Flowers

An extremely relaxing, almost sedating blend that makes one feel they are in a romantic Victorian garden on a hot summer night.

Rose	4 parts
Geranium	1 part
Eucalyptus	50 to 70 percent of blend

Chapter Five

The Application of Aromatherapy

The following is an index of health conditions and aromatic essential oils (EO's) which may be used in their treatment.

Important Notice

It is important to realize that this Therapeutic Index is not intended as a substitute for treatment by a qualified physician. Aromatherapy, in and by itself, cannot claim to be effective in the treatment, mitigation or alleviation of any condition. It is an effective 'adjunct' to other basic therapy modalities, especially clinical herbology and holistic based emotional healing, such as that found in hypnotherapy.

Why have I said "clinical herbology and holistic based emotional healing..." and not the other healing modalities (orthodox or otherwise)? Because here in America no other healing modalities have embraced aromatherapy to the extent that clinical herbalists and hypnotherapists have.

In Europe the story is different. Even the medical fraternity there widely recognizes and utilizes pure botanically derived EO's as therapeutic adjuncts in their treatments. But alas, this is America, home of the greatest medical dark age ever imposed by corporate driven special interests and political machinations upon a people. However, I see herbalism, especially clinical herbalism, and holistic hypnotherapy (and all its variations of emotional healing work) as the light at the end of this dark tunnel. Aromatherapy is proving to be a major part of this glowing hope for better answers and results.

A Word of Caution

Because of the idiosyncreatic (i.e. unpredicatble) nature of the individual and the fact that many health problems can't be simplistically ascertained, one must ever be aware that all conditions are multi-dimensional. The role of the healer must always take this into consideration, since life is seldom, if ever 'black-n-white." This means that someone simply saying they have a "belly ache" or a "headache" is inadequate, especially where deciding which aromatic essential oil to use is concerned. Be as thorough and complete in the assessment of a given condition as you can be, then determine, using the techniques described in Chapter 4, which EO's to use and how to use them.

A Promise Kept

As promised in the phrase, A User-Friendly Guide, found in the sub-title, this Therapeutic Index is easy to understand. After each condition I've listed EO's which may be helpful for that condition. I've italicized the aromatic essential oils that are the most proven to benefit that condition. For instructions on how to use the oils both internally and externally, please see Chapter 4, The Practice of Aromatherapy.

Where applicable I have also indicated appropriate key herbs which may be used in conjunction with the oils. Key herbs to take or use are listed inside the { } symbol. By 'key' herb, I mean to imply those single herbs which are most critical in treating a particular problem. Herbal combinations can also be selected using these key herbs. Simply look for formulas which list these key herbs as primary herbs in the formula (usually the first and/or second herb listed on the label). Except where noted otherwise these herbs are intended for internal use. Certain endangered herbs have been substituted with appropriate herbs.[9]

EO Warnings

Under pregnancy, hypertension and epilepsy are found lists of oils which SHOULD NOT be used in these conditions. In addition, the following oils begin to exhibit symptoms of toxicity when used internally in doses of ten drops or more: cinnamon, citronella, clove, fennel, lemon, nutmeg, pine and sage. Please do not use these oils internally in large quantities.

Therapeutic Index

-A-

ABCESS (COLD): *garlic*, cajeput. {burdock, echinacea, plantain}.

---

[9] Endangered herbs include golden seal and lady's slipper for which I've substituted barberry and valerian repsectively.

ABCESS (HOT): *clove*, lavender. {burdock, echinacea, plantain}.

ACNE: *cajeput*, juniper, lavender. (burdock, chaparral, juniper}.

AEORPHAGY (gulping air): *coriander*, fennel, lemon, *marjoram*, peppermint. {lobelia}.

ALBUMINURIA (high albumin in urine): *juniper*. {cedar berry, rose hips}.

ALOPECIA (hair loss on the head): lavender, *sage*, thyme. {ginseng, kelp, alfalfa}.

ANAL FISTULA (reoccurring anal abscess): *lavender*. {burdock, echinacea, collinsonia (stone root)}.

ANEMIA (low red blood cell count): chamomile, *garlic*, lemon. {yellow dock, nettles, dandelion, kelp}.

ANEMIA: (infantile): *thyme*. {yellow dock, purslaine}.

ANTISEPTICS: cinnamon, *eucalyptus*, garlic, juniper, *lavender, pine*, rosemary, *tea tree*, thyme. {garlic, herbal vinegars}.

ANXIETY (sympathetic): lavender, marjoram. {scullcap, valerian, kava kava, hops}.

ANXIETY (parasympathetic): thyme. {lobelia, valerian, kava kava}.

APHTHAE (oral and throat thrush): *geranium*, lemon, *sage*, tea tree. {garlic, clove}.

APPETITE (loss of – includes anorexia): bergamot, *chamomile, coriander*, fennel, garlic, ginger, juniper, lemon, nutmeg, sage. {slippery elm, chammomile, chickweed}.

APPETITE (over active): geranium, grapefruit, *lavender, marjoram.* {fennel, kava kava}.

ARTERIOSCLEROSIS: *garlic*, juniper, *lemon.* {horsetail, grape seed, rose hips}.

ARTHRITIS: garlic, *juniper, lemon*, thyme. {alfalfa, yellow dock, yucca, hydrochloric acid}.

ASTHMA: cajeput, eucalyptus, *garlic, lavender*, lemon, marjoram, peppermint, *pine, rosemary*, sage, tea tree, thyme. {lobelia, pluerisy root, scullcap}.

ATONIC DIGESTION: cinnamon, lavender, lemongrass, *sage.* {ginger, capsicum, fiber rich foods}

-B-

BAD BREATH (due to dyspepsia): lemon, *peppermint*, rosemary, thyme. {peppermint, pepsin, clove}.

BILIOUS ATTACK (swollen liver): peppermint. {catnip, slippery elm, fresh squeezed lemon in water}.

BI-POLAR CONDITION (manic/depression): *grapefruit.* {licorice, kava kava, St. John's Wort}.

BITES (animals): *clove*, lavender, *sage.* {echinacea, rose hips}.

BITES (reptiles and scorpians): clove, lavender, *sage.* {echinacea, rose hips}.

BITES & STINGS (insects and spiders*): cinnamon, lavender*, tea tree, thyme. {black cohosh, echinacea}.

BOILS: *chamomile*, lemon, thyme. {burdock, chaparral, garlic, poke root}.

BREAST CONGESTION: fennel, geranium, *rose.* {fenugreek, thyme, elder flowers}.

BRITTLENESS (hair and nails): *lemon*, peppermint. {horsetail, alfalfa, mullin}.

BRONCHIAL INFLUENZA: cinnamon, *clove, eucalyptus*, lemon, thyme. {fenugreek, thyme, garlic}.

BRONCHITIS (acute): cajeput*, eucalyptus*, garlic, *lavender*, lemon, *pine.* {lobelia, comfrey, ginger, uva ursi}.

BRONCHITIS (chronic): cajeput, *eucalyptus*, garlic, *lavender*, lemon, peppermint, pine, *rosemary*, sage, sandalwood, tea tree, thyme. {lobelia, fenugreek, rose hips}.

BURNS: *chamomile*, eucalyptus, geranium, *lavender*, rosemary, sage tea tree. {aloe vera, barberry, horsetail, white willow}.

-C-

CALMING EO's: cinnamon, pine, *lavender*, lemongrass, marjoram, patchouli, rose, sage.

CANCER (prevention and treatment of): clove, pine, garlic, *geranium*, sage. {burdock, red clover, chaparral, sage}.

The Application of Aromatherapy

CAPILLARY INSUFFICIENCY (fragile): *lemon,* peppermint. {blessed thistle, capsicum}.

CARDIAC FATIGUE: *garlic.* {hawthorn, garlic, angelica, shavegrass}.

CATARRH: cinnamon, *lemon,* marjoram, peppermint, thyme. {lobelia, fenugreek, plantain, ginger}.

CELLULITIS (painful): *grapefruit,* pine, marjoram.

CHAPPED SKIN: *rose.* {aloe vera & calendula used topically}.

CHILDBIRTH (preparing for, especially 5W before): *clove,* sage. {red raspberry, squaw vine, blessed thistle}.

CHILLS: *cinnamon,* ginger, thyme. {capsicum, ginger}.

CHOLECYSTITIS (gall bladder inflammation): pine, *rosemary.* {barberry, plantain, calendula}.

CHOLERA: *cinnamon,* eucalyptus, peppermint, sage, *tea tree.* (burdock, echinacea, barberry, garlic}.

CHOLESTEROL (high): *rosemary, thyme.* {shepherd's purse, grape seed}.

CICATRISING AGENTS (for rapid tissue healing w/minimal scaring): cajeput, chamomile, clove, eucalyptus, garlic, juniper, *lavender, rosemary, sage,* tea tree, thyme. {comfrey, aloe vera, slippery elm}.

CIRCULATORY DISORDERS (general): pine, *garlic,* lemon, thyme. {capsicum, ginger, passion flower}.

CIRRHOSIS: juniper, *rosemary.* {burdock, red clover}.

CLUSTER HEADACHES *(see headaches vaso-constrictive).*

COLIBACILLOSIS (E-coli infestation - colitis): eucalyptus, *sandalwood*, tea tree. {wild yam - comfrey - peach bark - barberry as a bolus}.

CONJUCTIVITIS: *chamomile*, lemon, rose. {barberry, calendula}.

CONSTIPATION (atonic): Coriander, *Garlic, Ginger*, Thyme. {capsicum, cascara sagrada, ginger, coarse fiber foods}.

CONSTIPATION (spastic): cardamom, *lavender*, *lemongrass*, marjoram. {flaxseed, fennel, soft fiber foods).

CONTAGIOUS DISEASES: cinnamon, *clove*, eucalyptus, *garlic*, ginger, juniper, *tea tree*. {barberry, garlic, echinacea, juniper}.

CONTUSIONS (bruises and bumps): *cinnamon*, clove, ginger, fennel, sage. {rose hips}.

CONVALESCENCE: *cardamom*, lemon, *sage*, thyme. {slippery elm, marshmallow, dandelion, licorice}.

CONVULSIONS: chamomile, lavender, *rose*. {chamomile, skunk cabbage, yarrow}.

COUGH (general): *eucalyptus*, fennel, tea tree. {Rose hips, yarrow, capsicum}.

COUGH (convulsive or spasmodic): eucalyptus, lavender, marjoram, *thyme*. {wild cherry bark, fenugreek}.

CYSTITIS (inflammations from cysts irritations): cajeput, eucalyptus, fennel, *juniper*, lavender, *pine*, sandalwood, tea tree, thyme. {burdock, echinacea}.

-D-

DEAFNESS (non-congenital): fennel, *garlic*. {mullein, plantain}.

DEBILITATION (general): *cardamom*, cinnamon, clove, eucalyptus, garlic, geranium, *ginger*, lavender, lemon, marjoram, nutmeg, *peppermint*, pine, *rosemary, sage,* tea tree, *thyme.* {slippery elm, marshmallow root, dandelion root}.

DEBILITATION (infantile): *lavender*, marjoram, *pine*, rosemary, sage. {slippery elm, marshmallow root}.

DEBILITATION (influenzal): *cinnamon*, lemon, sage, *tea tree*, thyme. {slippery elm, mistletoe}.

DECALCIFICATION: lemon. {alfalfa, comfrey, oatstraw}.

DEMINERALIZATION: *lemon* (calcium*), peppermint* (potassium). {irish moss, alfalfa liquid colloidal trace minerals}.

DEPRESSION (intermittent): *grapefruit*, lavender, thyme, bergamot. {ginko, gotu kola}.

DEPRESSION (chronic): *bergamot*, thyme. {St. John's Wort, gotu kola}.

DERMATOSIS (skin problems): cajeput, *chamomile*, *geranium*, juniper, sage, *tea tree*, thyme. {calendula, burdock}.

DIABETES: eucalyptus, *geranium, juniper*. {marsh mallow, dandelion, horsetail, kelp}.

DIARRHEA (general): chamomile, cinnamon, clove, garlic, geranium, ginger, juniper, *lavender*, lemon, nutmeg, peppermint, rosemary, sage, *sandalwood*, tea tree. {dandelion, red raspberry, comfrey}.

DIARRHEA (infantile): *chamomile*, sage. {red reaspberry, pumpkin seeds}.

DIARRHEA (tubercular): sage. {slippery elm, white oak bark, sun flower leaves (in the most serious cases)}.

DIPHTHERIA: *garlic*, tea tree, thyme. {barberry, clove buds, fenugreek, thyme}

DISINFECTANT (general houselhold): eucalyptus, juniper, lavender, sage, tea tree. {soaked solution of pine needles, clove bud, and sage}.

DISINFECTANT (public/institutional): eucalyptus, clove, pine, thyme. {soaked solution of pine needles, clove buds, and sage}.

DIURETICS: *grapefruit, juniper*, rosemary, sage. {juniper, marshmallow, corn silk, uva ursi, green matte}.

DROPSY (fluid retention in the lower body): garlic, *grapefruit, juniper*. {marshmallow, dandelion, corn silk, hydrangea, green matte}.

DYSPEPSIA (general): bergamot, *chamomile*, cinnamon, clove, *coriander*, fennel, garlic, *ginger*, juniper, lavender, *lemon, lemongrass*, peppermint, sage, thyme. {lemongrass, spearmint, thyme}.

DYSPEPSIA (atonic): bergamot, *cinnamon*, fennel, garlic, ginger, juniper, lavender, lemongrass, nutmeg, *peppermint*, rosemary, *sage, thyme.* {peppermint, ginger, chamomile}.

DYSPEPSIA (nervous): *coriander*, lavender, rose.

-E-

EARACHE: *cajeput*, garlic, *lavender.* {lobelia, mullein flowers}.

EAR INFLAMMATION (OTITIS): lemon, *lavender.* {mullein flowers, garlic}.

ECZEMA (general): *chamomile*, rose, sage. {burdock, juniper, kelp, plantain}.

ECZEMA (dry): *geranium*, lavender. {burdock, irish moss, plantain}.

ECZEMA (weeping): *juniper*, pine, *rose.* {burdock, marshmallow, plantain}.

EMMENAGOGUES: chamomile, cinnamon, fennel, juniper, lavender, nutmeg, peppermint, *rosemary, sage thyme.* {blue cohosh, black cohosh}.

EMPHYSEMA: eucalyptus, garlic, lavender, *thyme.* {comfrey, fenugreek, licorice}.

ENURESIS (bed wetting): *pine.* {bistort, corn silk, juniper, oat straw, uva ursi}.

EPIDEMICS (prevention of): eucalyptus, *garlic*, juniper *lemon*, pine, sandalwood. {garlic, burdock, echinacea}.

EPILEPSY: cajeput, *rosemary*, thyme. {black cohosh, lobelia} CAUTION: DO NOT use fennel or sage with epilepsy.

EYELIDS (inflammation): *chamomile*, lemon, rose. {eyebright, fennel, barberry root (as eyewash tissanes)}.

-F-

FACIAL NEURALGIA (tics): chamomile, *geranium, rose*. {the EO's mixed with a sprayable solution of aloe vera}.

FAINTING: *cinnamon*, garlic, rosemary. {ginko, gotu kola, ginger}.

FEBRILE STIFFNESS (stiffness caused by a fever): *lavender*, rose. {lobelia, fenugreek, hops}.

FEET (general irritations): lemon, pine, *rose*. {calendula, plantain}.

FEET (sweating, bad smelling): pine, *sage*, tea tree, *thyme*. {black walnut, sage}.

FEVERISH STATE (incoherent, delirious): eucalyptus, lemon, *sage*, tea tree. {catnip, gentain, yarrow, garlic}.

FEVERS (eruptive): eucalyptus, *lavender, rose*, tea tree. {yarrow, elder flowers, peppermint, corn silk}.

FLATULENCE: bergamot, chamomile, cinnamon, clove, *coriander, fennel*, garlic, *ginger*, lavender, lemon, marjoram, nutmeg, *peppermint*, rosemary, sage, thyme. {ginger, spearmint, caraway, papaya}.

FRECKLES: *lemon*, chamomile.

-G-

GALSTONES: *lemon*, nutmeg, pine, rosemary. {cascara sagrada, calendula}.

GASTRALGIA (general gastric pains): cinnamon, *fennel*, geranium peppermint, pine, *rose*, rosemary. {fennel, fenugreek}.

GASTRORRHAGIA (gastric hemorrhage): *lemon (taken with cayenne pepper)*. {capsicum, white oak bark}.

GINGIVITIS (common gum disease): *lemon*, sage, tea tree. {white oak & peach bark used as a mouth powder}.

GLANDULAR IMBALANCE: garlic, lemongrass, *rose*, sage. {damiana, ginseng, sarsaparilla, licorice}.

GOITER: *garlic, lemon*. {black walnut, kelp}.

GONORRHOEA: garlic, *lavender*, lemon, *sage, sandalwood*. {black walnut, barberry, yellow dock}.

GOUT: cajeput, chamomile, fennel, *garlic, juniper*, lemon, pine, *rosemary*, tea tree, thyme. {alfalfa, oat straw, horsetail, black walnut, hydrochloric acid}.

GUMS (to strengthen): fennel, *lemon*, sage, *tea tree*, thyme. {white oak bark, myrrh}.

-H-

HEMORRHOIDS: garlic, *lavender,* rose. {white oak bark, buckthorn, plantain, barberry, comfrey & peach bark as a bolus }.

HEMOPHILIA: lemon. {capsicum, dandelion, ginger}.

HAIR (general care): *rosemary,* thyme. {alfalfa, horsetail, kelp}.

HEADACHE (vaso-constrictive): *cardamom, lavender,* marjoram, peppermint. {white willow bark, peppermint, lavender blossoms}.

HEADACHE (vaso-dilative): grapefruit, *lemon.* (blessed thistle, eyebright, elder flowers, green matte, passion flower}.

HEMORRHAGE (internal): Cinnamon, *geranium,* rose. {capsicum, white oak bark, horsetail, calendula}.

HEMORRHAGE (external): rose, *geranium,* sandalwood. {capsicum, barberry}.

HEMORRHAGE (vaginal/uterine): Cinnamon, *geranium*, juniper, sandalwood. {marshmallow, mistletoe, red raspberry}.

HEPATIC CONGESTION: chamomile, *lemon, rosemary*, sage, thyme. {burdock, yellow dock, buckthorn}.

HEPATIC DEFICIENCY: *lemon.* {yellow dock, calendula, gentain}.

HEPATIC DISORDERS: lemon, peppermint, *rosemary, sage*, thyme. {burdock, echinacea, red clover}.

HERPES: chamomile, *geranium, grapefruit,* lemon. {barberry, black walnut, rose hips}.

HOOKWORM: thyme. {black walnut, horsetail}.

HYPERCOAGULATION OF BLOOD: garlic, *lemon.* {alfalfa, white willow bark, horsetail}.

HYPERTENSION (high blood pressure): *garlic,* lavender, lemon, *marjoram.* {garlic, gotu kola, lavender blossoms} CAUTION: DO NOT use rosemary, sage or thyme with hypertension.

HYPOTENSION (low blood pressure): rosemary, *sage,* thyme. {licorice, ginger, parsley, hawthorn}.

HYSTERIA (general): cajeput, chamomile, *lavender, rose,* rosemary. {hops, valerian, chamomile}.

-I-

IMPOTENCE: cinnamon, ginger, juniper, peppermint, *pine,* rosemary, *sandalwood,* thyme, ylang ylang. {saw palmetto, ginseng, shepherd's purse, licorice}.

INFECTIONS (various): All essences are to one degree or another bactericidal – especially cajeput, clove, eucalyptus, garlic, lavender, lemon, pine, tea tree and thyme. {barberry, echinacea}.

INFLUENZA: chamomile, *cinnamon, eucalyptus,* fennel, *garlic, lavender, lemon,* peppermint, *pine,* rosemary, sage, tea tree, *thyme.* {garlic, echinacea, barberry, clove bud, thyme}.

INSECT BITES & STINGS: *cinnamon*, garlic, *lavender*, lemon, sage, tea tree, thyme. {plantain}.

INSECT REPELLENT: clove, *citronella, lemongrass*, tea tree. {garlic, B vitamins}.

INTESTINAL COLIC: fennel, *bergamot*, peppermint. {catnip, fennel}.

INTESTINAL INFECTIONS (colitis, enteritis, etc.): bergamot, cajeput, chamomile, cinnamon, *garlic*, geranium, *lavender, lemongrass, rose*, rosemary, *thyme*, ylang ylang. {barberry, lavender blossoms, white oak bark}.

INTESTINAL PARASITES: *bergamot*, cajeput, chamomile, cinnamon, clove, eucalyptus, fennel, *garlic, lavender*, lemon, peppermint, tea tree, *thyme*. {black walnut, garlic, horsetail}.

IRRITABILITY (general): chamomile, lavender, *marjoram*. {catnip, chamomile, valerian}.

ITCHING (general): vinegar wash of *chamomile & rose*.

-J-

JAUNDICE: *geranium*, lemon, rosemary. {calendula, irish moss, oat straw, rose hips, yellow dock}.

-L-

LACTATION (to stimulate): *fennel*, lemongrass. {marshmallow, blessed thistle, fennel}.

LACTATION (to dry up): peppermint, *sage*. {sage, white oak bark}.

LARYNGITIS: *cajeput*, sage, tea tree. {gargle of red raspberry & lobelia tissane}.

LIBIDO (lack of): *cardamom*, cinnamon, *coriander*, sandalwood, *ylang ylang*. {male: saw palmetto, damiana; female: licorice, ginseng}.

LIBIDO (over stimulated): marjoram. {hops, valerian}.

LICE, TICS & CHIGGERS: *Cinnamon*, eucalyptus, clove, geranium, *lavender*, lemon, *lemongrass*, rosemary, *thyme*.

LUMBAGO (pain of the lower back): chamomile, *geranium*, juniper. {cascara sagrada, passion flower, white willow bark}.

LYMPHATISM (lymphatic congestion): *grapefruit*, lavender, rosemary, *sage*. {lobelia, mullein, plantain}.

-M-

MALARIA: clove, eucalyptus, lemon, *tea tree*. {fenugreek, echinacea}.

MEASLES: eucalyptus (diffused). {echinacea}.

MEMORY (loss of): clove, *coriander, rosemary*. {ginko, periwinkle, gotu kola}.

MENOPAUSE: chamomile, *geranium*, sage. {alfalfa, blessed thistle, damiana, kelp}.

MENSTRUATION (absence of): chamomile, peppermint, sage, *thyme*. {blue cohosh}.

MENSTRUATION (difficult and uncomfortable): *juniper*, lavender. {black cohosh}.

MENSTRUATION (painful): cajeput, *chamomile*, juniper, *peppermint*, rosemary, *sage.* (black cohosh}.

MENSTRUATION (scanty): cinnamon, *fennel*, lavender, *nutmeg*, peppermint, *sage.* {blue cohosh}.

MENTAL FATIGUE (from mental strain): clove, *rosemary*, thyme. {ginko, gotu kola}.

MENTAL INSTABILITY (thought disordered): *lemongrass*, marjoram, thyme. {kava kava, gotu kola, ginko}.

MIGRAINE (*see headache vaso-dilative*).

MOTION SICKNESS: *ginger*, lavender. {ginger}.

MOUTH INFLAMMATIONS: *geranium*, lemon, rose, sage. {white oak bark, peach bark}.

MUSCULAR STIFFNESS: *nutmeg*, rosemary, thyme, *rose*, {capsicum, lobelia, ginger, chamomile}.

-N-

NERVOUS DEBILITY: *coriander*, lavender, marjoram, *sage*, thyme. {chamomile, dandelion}.

NERVOUS STATES (ENERVATION): *lavender*, marjoram, rose. {chamomile, dandelion, lavender blossoms}.

NERVOUS SYSTEM (to balance): *lavender*, rosemary sage. {chamomile, lobelia, scullcap, valerian}.

NETTLE RASH (urticaria): *chamomile*, geranium. {aloe vera, eyebright}.

NOSEBLEED: chamomile, *lemon*. {washcloth drenched in a cold red raspberry & ginger iced tea then applied directly over nose, eyes and forehead}.

-O-

OBESITY: *fennel*, garlic, *grapefruit, lemon*. {uva ursi, parsley, cascara sagrada, oat straw}.

OEDEMA: *garlic*, geranium, rose. {uva ursi, parsley, plantain, juniper, mullein}.

OPHTHALMIA (general eye problems): *chamomile*, geranium, rose. {eyebright, horsetail, alfalfa}.

OVARIES (ovarian problems): geranium, *sage*. {blessed thistle, red raspberry}.

OXYURIS (pin-worm, threadworm, etc.): *chamomile*, eucalyptus, *garlic*, lemon, thyme. {black walnut, horsetail}.

-P-

PALPITATIONS: lemongrass, *peppermint*, rosemary. {lobelia, hawthorn}.

PANCREATIC DEFICIENCY: juniper, *lemon, peppermint*. {licorice, elecampane}.

PARALYSIS (general): *peppermint*, sage. {slippery elm, ginko, gotu kola, horsetail}.

PARALYSIS (after-effects of): *juniper*, lavender, *pine*, rosemary. {alfalfa, ginko, gotu kola, horsetail, blessed thistle}.

PNEUMONIA: *eucalyptus*, lavender, lemon, *pine*. {comfrey, fenugreek, lobelia, pleurisy root}.

POISONING (gastro-intestinal): *peppermint*, cinnamon, lavender, tea tree. {vinegar of lobelia – clove bud – thyme}.

PREGNANCY – CAUTION: do not use the following during pregnancy: clove, juniper, marjoram, nutmeg, peppermint, rosemary and sage.

PROSTATITIS (inflammation of): pine, *sandalwood*. {marsh mallow, corn silk, black walnut, uva ursa}.

PSORIASIS: cajeput, *lavender*. {calendula, burdock}.

PUBERTY: garlic, *pine*, thyme. {damiana, ginseng, licorice}.

PULMONARY DISEASES: cajeput, clove, eucalyptus, fennel, *garlic*, lavender, lemon, peppermint, *pine*, sage, *sandalwood*, *tea tree*, thyme. {mullein, garlic, fenugreek}.

PULMONARY EMPHYSEMA: *garlic*, tea tree, *thyme*. {lobelia, fenugreek, mullein, garlic}.

PULMONARY GANGRENE: eucalyptus, *garlic, tea tree*. (mullein, plantain, fenugreek}.

PULMONARY TUBERCULOSIS: cajeput, clove, *eucalyptus*, garlic, lavender, *lemon*, peppermint, *pine*, sage, thyme. {fenugreek, thyme, clove bud}.

PURIFICATION OF DRINKING WATER: *lemon*, tea tree. {squeeze 1/2 fresh lemon per 16 oz water and let peel sit in water for 5 minutes before drinking}.

PUTREFACTIVE FERMENTATION (improper protein digestion): cinnamon, *clove*, ginger, juniper, *thyme*. {ginger, clove bud, hydrochloric acid}.

-R-

RESPIRATORY DEFICIENCY: cinnamon, *garlic*. {mullin, lobelia, fenugreek}.

RHEUMATIC PAINS: *cajeput*, chamomile, *coriander, eucalyptus*, garlic, ginger, lavender, marjoram, *nutmeg*. {yellow dock, white willow bark, horsetail, hydrochloric acid}.

RHEUMATISM (chronic): *cajeput*, chamomile, *eucalyptus, garlic*, juniper, lavender, lemon, pine, rosemary *thyme*. {brigham tea, burdock, elder flowers}.

RHEUMATISM (muscular): marjoram, *rosemary*, thyme. {brigham tea, sage, yarrow}.

RHINITIS (sinus infections): tea tree, *thyme*. {fenugreek, barberry}.

ROUNDWORM (ringworm): chamomile, eucalyptus, garlic, *tea tree, thyme*. {black walnut, pumpkin seed}.

-S-

SCABIES (skin parasite): *cinnamon*, clove, garlic, *lavender*, lemon, peppermint, pine rosemary, *tea tree*, thyme. {black walnut, garlic}.

SCARLET FEVER: *eucalyptus*, tea tree (diffused). {brigham tea, echinacea, bayberry, hawthorn, yarrow}.

SCROFULOSIS: garlic, lavender, *sage*. {black walnut, garlic, horsetail}.

SCURVY: *lemon, garlic*, ginger (with fresh lime or lemon water).

SEDATIVES: *chamomile, lavender*, lemon, *marjoram*, nutmeg, thyme. {lobelia, hops, valerian}.

SENESCENCE (mental wanderings due to aging): garlic, *lemon, thyme*. {ginko, gotu kola, lecithin}.

SHINGLES: geranium. {valerian, scullcap}.

SHOCK (nervous crisis): chamomile, *lavender, rose*. {capsicum & lobelia, hops, ginger, scullcap, lavender flowers, valerian}.

SIGHT (poor or weak): rosemary. {eyebright, fennel}.

SINUSITIS (inflamed sinuses): eucalyptus, lavender, lemon, peppermint, *pine*, tea tree, *thyme*. {comfrey, fenugreek, elder flowers, bayberry}.

SMOKING: coriander, *sage*. {lobelia, valerian}.

SNAKE BITES (including Gila Monsters): anti-venom blend of *cinnamon, lavender*, lemon, thyme. {plantain, lavender blossoms}.

SPASMS (general):*coriander*, lavender, marjoram. {lobelia, wild lettuce, wild yam}

SPASMS (cardiac): lemongrass. {lobelia, hawthorn, lemongrass}.

SPASMS (gastric): *cajeput*, peppermint. {spearmint, catnip, chamomile, wild yam}.

SPASMS (intestinal): *bergamot*, cajeput, *chamomile*. cinnamon, clove, fennel, garlic lavender, peppermint, pine. {chamomile, fennel seed, licorice}.

SPASMS (vascular): garlic. {lobelia, hawthorn, valerian}.

SPERMATORRHOEA: lavender, *marjoram*. {flax seed, saw palmetto, black walnut}.

STIMULANTS (adrenal cortex): *geranium*, pine, rosemary, sage. {licorice}.

STIMULANTS (cardiac): rosemary, *ylang ylang*. (hawthorne, capsicum}.

STIMULANTS (circulatory and respiratory): *cinnamon*, tea tree. {hawthorne, thyme}

STIMULANTS (nervous system): *cardamom*, rosemary, sage. {ginger, horseraddish}.

SWEATING (profuse): sage, thyme. {elder flowers}.

SYMPATHETIC NERVOUS (dystonia of): *lemongrass*, marjoram, rosemary. {passion flower, oat straw, fennel}.

SYPHILIS: lemon. {yellow dock, parsley, black walnut}.

SYPHILITIC SORES: *lavender*, rose. {yellow dock, black walnut, fenugreek}.

-T-

TACHYCARDIA (irregular heart beat): garlic, pine, *ylang ylang*. {garlic, hawthorn, valerian}.

TAPEWORM: garlic, thyme. {garlic, horsetail, black walnut}.

TEETH CARE: *clove*, lemon, peppermint, *thyme*. (alfalfa, oat straw, horsetail}

TEETHING: *chamomile*, lavender, clove. {slippery elm or marsh mallow stick to chew on}.

THROAT (general soreness): *geranium*, ginger, *lemon*, sage, *thyme*. {fenugreek, comfrey, thyme}.

TONSILLITIS: *geranium*, ginger, lemon, sage, *tea tree, thyme*. {fenugreek, thyme, clove, slippery elm}.

TOOTHACHE: cajeput, cinnamon, *clove*, garlic, juniper, *nutmeg*, peppermint, sage. {clove, lobelia, white willow bark}.

TREMORS (palsy like conditions): peppermint, *marjoram*, rosemary, sage. {lobelia, blue cohosh, wild yam}.

TYPHOID FEVER: cinnamon, garlic, lavender, *lemon, thyme*. (barberry, black cohosh).

TYPHUS: eucalyptus, *tea tree*. {garlic, burdock, echinacea}.

-U-

ULCERS (stomach and gastro-intestinal) *Chamomile, geranium*, lemon, rose. {gentain, cyani flowers, dandelion, chaparral}.

URETHRITIS (inflammation of the urinary tract): cajeput. {peach bark, marsh mallow, corn silk}.

URIC ACID (excess): lemon. {alfalfa, blessed thistle}.

URINARY INFECTIONS: cajeput, eucalyptus, fennel, geranium, lavender, lemon, pine, sage, *sandalwood, thyme.* {uva ursi, cornsilk, barberry}.

URINARY STONES: fennel, garlic, geranium, lemon. {queen of the meadow, marsh mallow, cornsilk}.

-V-

VAGINAL DISCHARGE: cinnamon, juniper, *lavender*, rosemary, *sage*, tea tree, thyme. {red raspberry, blessed thistle}.

VARICOSE VEINS: garlic, *juniper*, lemon. {white oak bark, horsetail, oat straw}.

VERTIGO (fear of heights, dizziness): chamomile, *lavender*, peppermint, *rosemary*, sage, thyme. {ginger}.

VOICE (loss of): lemon, thyme. {gargle of vinegar w/fenugreek}.

VOMITING (general): lemon, *peppermint*. {ginger, licorice}.

VOMITING (nervous): cajeput, *fennel*, peppermint. {ginger, fennel}.

-W-

WARTS: *clove, garlic*, lemon. {garlic, chaparral, black walnut}.

WHOOPING COUGH: *garlic, lavender*, marjoram, rosemary, thyme. {fenugreek, garlic, thyme}.

WOUNDS (atonic, ulcerated, etc.): cajeput, *clove, garlic, juniper*, lavender, rosemary, *sage, tea tree, thyme,* {poultice of myrrh, - barberry - plantain}.

WOUNDS (infected): Cajeput, *chamomile, clove, eucalyptus, garlic, lavender*, rosemary, *tea tree.* {poultice of plantain – comfrey – queen of the meadow - barberry}.

WOUNDS, SORES & CUTS: cajeput, *chamomile,* clove, *eucalyptus*, garlic, geranium, juniper *lavender*, rosemary, sage, *tea tree*, thyme. {burdock, echinacea, barberry}.

WRINKLES: *grapefruit, patchouli*, lemon. {calendula, aloe vera}.

-Y-

YEAST INFECTIONS (candida, etc.): clove, garlic, lavender, *sandalwood*, tea tree, *thyme.* {garlic, barberry, burdock, echinacea, chaparral, pau d' arco}.

Getting Started – The Most Important Step

Now, what you'll need to do is get yourself a starter kit. I recommend the following as a viable starter kit that will take care of most personal, household and family needs in a pinch. Lemon, Lavender, Eucalyptus, Tea Tree, Pine, Peppermint and Thyme. To that add a small container of Almond oil and a small porcelain mixing plate (i.e. a small 2 inch by 1/2 inch deep oriental dipping sauce bowl) to mix the EO's and almond oil in. For those more adventurous, try some hemp oil cut with grape seed oil to which you've added the specific EO's your planning on using.

Once you've compiled your basic starter kit and begin to add other EO's, the next step is to get a good quality nebulizing diffuser.

A nebulizing diffuser uses a small aquarium sized pump to blow air into a glass nebulizer. The air goes into a small chamber that causes a pressure back-draft and pulls the EO's up a small tube. As the EO's come to the top of the tube the air flow catches the EO's blows them against the wall of the glass which causes the EO's to hit with such force that the EO's molecule chains are smashed into smaller and smaller molecule chains until they become lighter than the surrounding air. The air going into the diffuser pushes the small molecules out into the air where the EO's then waft through the room doing all their good.

Due to their extensive use of and concurrent developments, the French have designed the best and most efficient nebulizing diffusers in the market. Like aromatic essential oils, nebulizing diffusers are no different, you really do get what you pay for.

It is essential that you use eucalyptus as the cutting oil for the diffuser, so you're going to need a bit more of it than other EO's if your planning on using a nebulizing diffuser.

Don't apply heat to EO's to diffuse them (similar to the cheap light bulb units found in dime stores and bargain magazines) as this will completely render the therapeutic benefits of EO's useless. Furthermore, heat diffusing can so change the molecular makeup of an EO that it now becomes an airborne allergin. Something it previously was not.

In Closing

I've presented this guide to you the way I have on the premise that it would make your usage of EO's a much more 'user-friendly' experience. The ramifications of formulating and blending EO's into consumer based products has been discussed, and as you have seen is a very involved process. Always remember the *Criteria & Standards for Using EO's* I introduced you to in Chapter 3 when purchasing and using EO's. You have been introduced to a number of the most consumer available pure botanically derived single EO's, their uses, unique healing properties, and their overall effect on neurological responses relative to their physiological and emotional effects. Both the professional and lay person should benefit from what's been presented. I hope my own personal observations and suggestions (many based on my own clinical experiences) on their uses and how to do some of your own simple blends is beneficial.

To get more out of your experience of aromatherapy you'll need to talk to others about it. Exchange information and collaborate on your experiences. Because it was so new I didn't have that advantage when I started out. Today the picture is different as more people are involved and the picture is more panoramic. Get a group of like-minded professional associates or individuals together who share the same concerns and

aspirations for greater health and wellbeing, and then share the wonderous, exotic and sensuous world of aromatic essential oils among yourselves and any others wanting the same. Start with a few neighbors, family, friends or working associates who share the same mindset as you, then let it grow from there.

Now take your favorite EO, open it and take a whiff of it. No, not a long knock out breath. Just put it a couple inches from the nose and lightly breath the aroma and let it waft into your nostrils. Ahhh... Isn't that nice? Feeling and healing good. That's what aromatic essential oils are all about. Enjoy.

Index

Index

The Scents of Health